Community Midwifery Practice

Community
Midwifery Practice

Edited by

**Jenny Edwins MSc, PGDip,
ADM/DPSM, SCM, RGN, OND**

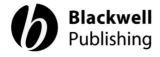

Blackwell
Publishing

Library of Congress Cataloging-in-Publication Data

Community midwifery practice / edited by Jenny Edwins.
p. ; cm.
Includes bibliographical references and index.
ISBN-13: 978-1-4051-4895-5 (pbk. : alk. paper)
ISBN-10: 1-4051-4895-0 (pbk. : alk. paper)   1. Midwifery.   2. Community
health services.   I. Edwins, Jenny.
[DNLM: 1. Midwifery–methods.   2. Community Health
Services–methods. WQ 160 C734 2008]
RG950.C62 2008
618.2–dc22
2007039585

A catalogue record for this book is available from the British Library.

Set in 10/12 pt Palatino by SNP Best-set Typesetter Ltd., Hong Kong
Printed in Singapore by Utopia Press Pte Ltd
1 2008

Contents

Contributors

Susan Blackburn BSc (Hons), RM
Independent midwife

Ann Bradshaw BSc (Hons), DipHE in Antenatal Education
NHS Parent Education Consultant and independent childbirth educator

Judy Byrne RGN, RM
Senior Midwife Manager, Worcestershire Acute Hospitals NHS Trust
and Supervisor of Midwives

Jean Chapple MBChB, MCommH, FFPH, FRCP, MFFP, DRCOG,
DCH
Programme Director, Westminster Primary Care Trust, Regional Child
Health Screening Coordinator for London

Jenny Edwins MSc, PGDip, ADM/DPSM, SCM, RGN, OND
Senior Lecturer in Midwifery, University of Worcester

Dianne Garland MSc, PGCEA, ADM, RM, SRN
Freelance and bank midwife, Governace Chair for Waterbirth
International

Ruth Jones MA, BA (Hons), Dip.NN
Lecturer in Sociology at the University of Worcester, trainer for Amnesty
International and member of the Women's National Commission –
Department of Trade and Industry, HEVAN (Health Ending Violence and
Abuse Now) and Women's Aid Federation of England

Elaine Newell BSc Hons (Midwifery), DPSM, RM, RN
Head of Midwifery, Worcestershire Acute Hospitals NHS Trust

Caroline Payne BSc (Hons), ENB 405, RM, RGN
Clinical Midwife and Infant Feeding Coordinator, Worcestershire Acute
Hospitals NHS Trust

Nadia Permalloo RM, RGN
Regional Antenatal Screening Coordinator for London

Carolyn Roth MSc, PGCEA, RM, RN
Lead Midwife for Education, Keele University

Kim Russell MA, PGCert HE, BSc (Hons), Cert. Health Ed. (Disc), RM,
RGN
Senior Lecturer in Midwifery, University of Worcester

Sarah Snow MSc, DPSM/ADM, BSc (Hons), C&G teaching certificate,
RM, RN
Senior Lecturer in Midwifery, University of Worcester

Judith Sunderland MSc, BSc (Hons), RM, RGN
Lecturer in Midwifery, City University (formerly HIV Specialist Midwife,
Newham University NHS Trust)

Preface

The idea for this book arose from informal discussions with clinical midwives, highlighting the fact that those who are new to practising in the community setting have to make a leap that involves a huge learning curve. The majority of midwives are eager to prepare themselves for a role that differs dramatically from that of a hospital-based practitioner but may not feel well equipped for this diverse experience. It has also been a long time since the publication of Cronk and Flint's (1990) much valued practical guide for community midwives. The clinical topics explored by Cronk and Flint are still of relevance but the current role of the community midwife is ever expanding. Many new publications are addressing the public health aspects of midwifery practice driven by the *National Service Framework for Children, Young People and Maternity Services* (DH, 2004) but this has to be underpinned by the clinical aspects of midwifery care that are the cornerstone of the profession.

This book aims to explore a number of topics within the context of current-day clinical midwifery practice in the community and there are numerous challenges. An increasing number of women are choosing birth at home and this is set to rise in the future with the introduction of 'choice guarantees'. Women with complex problems, such as pelvic girdle pain or a diagnosis of HIV infection, must have their needs met effectively and women living with domestic abuse need to have the question asked.

It is hoped that each chapter will act as a resource to support practitioners in their goal to deliver women-centred care. Judy Byrne encapsulated the aim of this book perfectly when she reflected on her own chapter to state that she wished somebody had written something similar for her to refer to when she was just beginning to work in the field of safeguarding children.

The chapters are diverse but one overall theme dominates: communication is fundamental to the role of the community midwife and she or he has the opportunity to connect with women every day and over time. But the pace of change and the constraints of an ever-increasing workload are a threat that can undermine the relationship between health professionals and the women in their care. Mary Field Belenky's quote reminds us of the importance of maintaining good communication – without it there is no relationship.

> 'Really listening and suspending one's own judgment is necessary in order to understand other people on their own terms . . . This is a process that requires trust and builds trust.' Mary Field Belenky (1997)

References

Belenky, M.F. (1997) *Women's Ways of Knowing: The Development of Self, Voice and Mind*. Basic Books, New York.

Cronk, M. and Flint, C. (1990) *Community Midwifery: A Practical Guide*. Butterworth-Heinemann, Oxford.

DH (2004) *National Service Framework for Children, Young People and Maternity Services*. Department of Health/Department for Education and Skills, London.

Acknowledgements

Health professionals are very busy people so my thanks to the contributing authors are heart felt. You have each done a great job in writing a chapter on top of your usual workload.

You learn a lot about human nature when you undertake a project like this and it's mostly good. I would like to thank everyone who helped me to source information, verify facts and grant permission to reproduce information.

Special thanks go to Louise Jones and my colleagues at the University of Worcester for their support. Those of you who took time out to read and comment on preliminary chapters were particularly helpful.

And last, but certainly not least, big thanks are due to Alex Clabburn for his unending patience and to Dave Jeffery for more than a little inspiration.

Jenny Edwins
August 2007

Introduction: ways of working in the community

Jenny Edwins

The primary source of job satisfaction for midwives working in the community involves building and maintaining an ongoing professional relationship with a woman and her family. Many community midwives must agree with this opening statement because it is relatively rare for them to return to working within a consultant-led unit: they become rooted in their patch, like trees. A role in the community is sometimes viewed by colleagues in the confines of the hospital environment as an isolating task. Some come out to give it a try and then return to the hospital base when they begin to miss the team. But how could a midwife be lonely working in the community setting? There is always a team around; they are just a little bit more distant in the physical sense.

Community midwives work with women in their own homes, gaining valuable insights into their social networks. The potential to connect with women over an extended period of time is a privilege. Hunter's study (2004) describes the significance of the community midwife's relationship with mothers as a source of emotional reward that transpires as job satisfaction. In contrast, she found that hospital-based midwives derived emotional reward from their relationships with colleagues and completion of the tasks associated with seeing women safely through the experience of giving birth and going home.

It would be impossible to avoid drawing on personal experience of working as a community midwife over a period of 13 years and a reflection from that time will open this chapter and close it. The chapter will then progress to consider some of the changes made to the organisation of maternity services in recent decades and how these have shaped the role of the community midwife in the UK. An exploration of current and future influences will follow, with particular reference to key policy documents.

Reflection

The patch that I covered from 1983 until 1996 included the semi-rural area that I was brought up in. An extended family of Romany travellers lived on a permanent site in this area, next to a ford that fills up rapidly in bad weather. My relationship with the childbearing women on the site took a long time to progress from that of tentative interaction to begin with, to one of negotiated trust over time. I had to learn to understand how this particular group of women viewed local health and social services and how they accessed these services on their own particular terms. It took a while to develop insight into a group of individuals from a different cultural background who had generally inherited a healthy distrust of all things official. As we got to know each other I was pleased to meet these women when they came to my antenatal clinic. Their confidence in me grew and, as a result, they increasingly shared their confidences with me.

Strict adherence to residential boundaries at the time meant that some of the women lived outside the GP catchment area, but these women wanted to be under the care of a particular female doctor and a familiar midwife. They therefore registered at the local practice using their mother's site address and hopped into their cars to travel over the geographical boundary to grandmother's van for postnatal visits and follow-up care from the health visitor.

These traveller women had distinct expectations that didn't always match those of health professionals. In fact, they achieved choice, continuity and a great degree of control over their care way before *Changing Childbirth* (DH, 1993) put in an appearance, but a number of my colleagues in the multidisciplinary team viewed this group of women as a challenge because they were 'non compliant'.

An equal relationship, based on partnership, facilitates a deeper knowledge of a woman's beliefs, aspirations and cultural perspectives. It therefore seems logical to state that the rhetoric of woman-centred care, within the context of her extended family and social support networks, is much more realisable in a community-based role that offers continuity over time, from one pregnancy to the next. Compare the opportunities to build continuing relationships that midwives working in the community have with those of colleagues working within the 'conveyer belt' system of many large consultant units and the former clearly have a great advantage.

Building a therapeutic relationship that goes some way towards equalising the power imbalance between professionals and service users is desirable for all women, but evidence suggests that this is less likely for women from minority groups. Lewis (2001, 2004) has highlighted the over-representation of such groups in recent *Confidential*

Enquiries into Maternal Deaths (CEMD). It has also been suggested by Khan and Pillay (2003) that the majority of nurses (and other health professionals by implication) are poorly prepared to work within a multicultural community. Khan and Pillay's stance indicates that health professionals trained in the UK have historically viewed differences in ethnicity and culture as a problem that needs to be solved by making changes to modify attitudes and induce conformity within the prevailing system. A more appropriate strategy would include reflection upon the practitioner's personal beliefs and identification of a client's needs, to incorporate cultural differences within a mutually devised plan of care.

Hindley (2005) describes her study, which explored the experiences of ethnic minority women in an inner city area with high levels of health-related and social need. It is interesting to note that this study was generated and funded from within the community as a direct result of women's dissatisfaction with existing maternity services. The overriding conclusion was that continuity of midwife carer matters greatly because continuity enables women to address inequalities in power. In turn, this greatly reduces the likelihood of prejudice or stereotyping. Hindley (2005) recommends a case-loading approach, based in the community, with a maximum of four midwives being involved in a woman's care. This fits very well into the current agenda driven by the CEMD to improve services for all women, but minority groups and the socially excluded in particular (Lewis, 2004).

Maternity services have consistently been shaped by government reports and policy and the *National Service Framework (NSF) for Children, Young People and Maternity Services* (DH, 2004) and the recent *Maternity Matters* document (DH/PCFM, 2007) suggest a significant general move towards community-focused delivery of care in the future. Community-based models have tremendous potential to facilitate services that individualise care to meet health and social needs, and to promote normal birth at a time when the caesarean section rate in the UK has risen to an all-time high in many areas.

A review of ways in which community midwives have worked in the past and a longer deliberation about current initiatives and how community midwifery services might be shaped in the future will follow.

The past

When the National Health Service (NHS) came into being in 1948, 'domiciliary' midwives were employed by local authorities to provide midwifery care in the community. As successive government reports (Ministry of Health, 1959; Standing Maternity and Midwifery Advisory Committee, 1970) drove birth from the home into hospital and GP units, the domiciliary midwives' scope of practice became more and more limited because they were only licensed to care for women giving birth in their own homes. This restriction hampered the development of integrated GP units up until the reorganisation of the NHS in 1974 (Campbell and Macfarlane, 1994). Midwives were then brought together to be employed wholesale by health authorities. The home birth rate subsequently continued to fall as official perceptions shaped the dominant view that hospital birth was the safest option for women and their babies. Munro (1984) summarised this perspective in the foreword of *Maternity Care in Action*, stating that 'the present practice whereby practically all mothers have their babies in hospital should continue to be promoted in the interests of the safety and welfare of the mother and her baby'. Both health professionals and consumers of the maternity services were influenced by the succession of three *Maternity Care in Action* reports that were largely based on opinion rather than evidence. As the 1980s unfolded, community midwives found that they were able to continue to provide ante- and postnatal care but a gap in continuity appeared as the great majority of women went into hospital to give birth. Many GPs withdrew their support for GP units as a result of *Maternity Care in Action*, leading to the closure of these popular units and diminished choice for women with low-risk pregnancies. It also became increasingly difficult to find a GP willing to provide medical cover for births at home and there were numerous distressing incidents whereby women were removed from GP lists when they tried to pursue the option of birth at home. The proportion of home births plummeted and many midwives began to lose their skills of watchful waiting in a woman's own home.

The publication of *Changing Childbirth* (DH, 1993) countenanced what many mothers and midwives had been calling for over a number of years. The report's mantra of choice, continuity and control was governed by the overriding principle of woman-centred care, veering significantly away from the paternalistic approach of previous policy documents. This exciting publication fuelled enthusiasm for the implementation of team midwifery projects as a vehicle for achieving many of the proposed 'ten indicators of success' and the future looked bright. The key indicators setting targets for pilot team midwifery projects were as follows:

- Every woman should know one midwife who ensures continuity of her midwifery care – the named midwife.
- At least 30% of women should have the midwife as lead professional.
- Every woman should know the lead professional who has a key role in the planning and provision of her care.
- At least 75% of women should know the person who cares for them during their delivery.
  (DH, 1993)

Some pilot team projects, largely based on the concept pioneered by Flint (1986), were already up and running but *Changing Childbirth* provided added impetus to boost their numbers across the UK. Wraight et al. (1993) clarified the level of provision of team midwifery services in their mapping exercise for the Department of Health (DH). Their survey of 269 maternity units in England and Wales elicited a 95% response and concluded that 100 units had established teams and 22 were piloting them. Despite the fact that a quarter of team midwifery schemes launched in 1990 had ceased within 12 months, Wraight et al. (1993) identified that 98 units had plans to implement similar projects. This indicates that a majority of maternity service providers supported the idea of team midwifery in principle.

Amongst a number of others, a study by Tinkler and Quinney (1998) identified women's perceptions of this type of care, to support the concept of team midwifery as an excellent means of meeting their needs. The opportunities to develop trusting relationships were reflected in high levels of satisfaction with the care provided. However, despite the demonstrable benefits for women, as further evaluations of team projects emerged their sustainability began to be questioned as high levels of midwife 'burnout' were identified as a major problem (Sandall, 1997; Barber, 1998). In addition, there is a view that the majority of projects were doomed to failure due to the limited amount of central funding made available to support the implementation of *Changing Childbirth* initiatives. Declercq (1998) describes the budget assigned to the Changing Childbirth Implementation Team as 'modest'. A pattern subsequently began to emerge and, despite excellent outcomes and glowing evaluations, many team schemes were abruptly discontinued.

There is no doubt that *Changing Childbirth* was the precursor to a movement towards a woman-centred service, with greater emphasis on equal partnerships in maternity care. Valiant efforts to implement and sustain team systems of care were apparent and the advantages in terms of delivering an excellent service to defined case-loads of particular women are clear. Modifications to the blueprint for the implementation of teams have been suggested through adjusting the emphasis on continuity of *carer* to continuity of *care* (Hicks et al., 2003) but, despite this, only a small number of community-based team midwifery projects are ongoing.

In summary, it is tempting to conclude that *Changing Childbirth* failed to deliver significant changes in relation to the reorganisation of maternity services. It did, however, initiate a veritable sea change in attitudes to firmly cement the ethos of woman-centred care and must be viewed as a significant document that continues to underpin current policy.

The National Service Framework and the future

The consultation document *A First Class Service* (DH, 1998) heralded the New Labour government's 10-year plan for modernisation of the NHS. It was followed in 2000 by the launch of *The NHS Plan* (DH, 2000), which reinforced priorities, including strong clinical governance, robust performance frameworks and consumer involvement in planning service provision. These global documents had very little for grass roots midwives to engage with specifically and it was some time before the publication of *Delivering the Best: Midwives Contribution to the NHS Plan* (DH, 2003) with its pointers for the development of maternity services. Quality issues were broken down to emphasise the use of evidence-based practice and best practice, and the important issue of leadership highlighted as an area for development. *Delivering the Best* was very successful in conveying a key message:

> 'The midwifery workforce of the twenty first century needs to develop to engage with issues of public health and multidisciplinary working.' DH (2003)

In view of the fact that maternity services have historically been shaped by government reports, it is appropriate for midwives to be aware of key DH publications, and the NSF (DH, 2004) in particular. The NSF for Children, Young People and Maternity Services is now firmly in place and Standard 11 of the document relates to maternity services. This chapter will continue to consider what Standard 11 might mean for midwives working in the community through the exploration of a number of issues.

The Albany Midwifery Practice

A straw poll of midwives suggests that policy documents such as the NSF and the excellent examples of successful initiatives in *Delivering the Best* have not been accessed widely by clinicians. Hart and Lockey (2002) agree that knowledge of current policy may be limited amongst practising midwives. As a body, midwives are much more likely to be aware of clinically based initiatives, such as the Albany Practice who are meeting the benchmarks of many aspects of Standard 11 of the NSF almost by default due to their adoption of a case-loading system of working.

Many authors support the assertion that continuity of carer improves outcomes for mothers and babies (Sandall et al., 2001; Hodnett, 2004). The Albany Midwifery Practice has consistently demonstrated a positive impact upon outcomes that include qualitative aspects such as satisfaction with care. After describing their results as spectacular, Rosser (2003) asks the question that must be on the mind of many midwives – how does the Albany Practice do it?

A group of independent midwives formed the South-East London Midwifery Group Practice in 1994 as a pilot project, driven by *Changing Childbirth* and its focus on improving continuity of care and carer (Reid, 2002a). Due to emerging funding difficulties they subcontracted their services to Kings Healthcare Trust in 1997, as the Albany Practice. They are now located, as one of nine group practices within the trust, in an inner city area with a high level of social deprivation. They care for both high- and low-risk women. Reid (2003b) describes how organisation is the key to ensuring excellent continuity of care. Each midwife has 12 weeks' holiday a year. Forward planning takes this into consideration when allocating case-loads so that primary midwives will be working when the women that they have cared for antenatally are due to give birth. The realities of living with a pager 24 hours a day are explored and rationalised. Women are given clear information regarding when to call the midwife out of office hours and as a result the midwives are rarely contacted at night for non-urgent advice. Naturally, the exceptions are women who are in labour and, in 2006, 46% of women gave birth to their babies at home (Armstrong, personal communication). On average, a midwife carrying a full case-load will be present at two births each week (Reid, 2003b). Outcomes are enviable, with high rates of normal birth and initiation of breastfeeding. The Albany midwives attribute this to their philosophy of 'a pattern of care in which a woman is attended during her pregnancy, labour and postnatal period by a midwife with whom a relationship of trust has been established' (Rosser, 2003).

It is clear that midwives currently working within a case-load system are self-selected. They share a common philosophy but this way of working also has to fit in with their lifestyle. Society has changed dramatically since the days of domiciliary midwifery and many midwives are now considering the need to achieve a healthy balance between a career and a family life. Case-loading may not be an option for some, but it is too easy to presume that this way of working would not be considered by a significant number of midwives. Retention of skilled midwifery staff is a continuing problem due to high levels of dissatisfaction with the current organisation of maternity services and the prevailing culture within the NHS (Ball et al., 2002; Curtis et al., 2006). The NSF offers opportunities to introduce new ways of working and case-loading is arguably the only model for consideration on the table at present.

One Mother One Midwife

The Independent Midwives Association has surveyed midwives to assess the feasibility of their proposal, known as the One Mother One Midwife (OMOM) campaign (Francis and Van der Kooy, 2004). They have developed a model that aims to address the barriers preventing the widespread adoption of a case-loading approach across the UK. The model proposes the implementation of a national contract that would allow primary healthcare trusts (PCTs) to extend the range of maternity services that they currently commission. Funding would be allocated to the NHS Community Midwifery Model (NHSCMM) and PCTs would have the option to employ midwives who would, in turn, be paid for each episode of pregnancy, birth and postnatal care. The money would follow the woman and this approach dovetails with the move towards payment by results within the NHS overall.

Some of the NHSCMM funding would be used to indemnify midwives opting to carry a self-determined case-load, through the NHS Litigation Authority (NHSLA). Midwives would naturally continue to be accountable for their own practice (Figure 1.1).

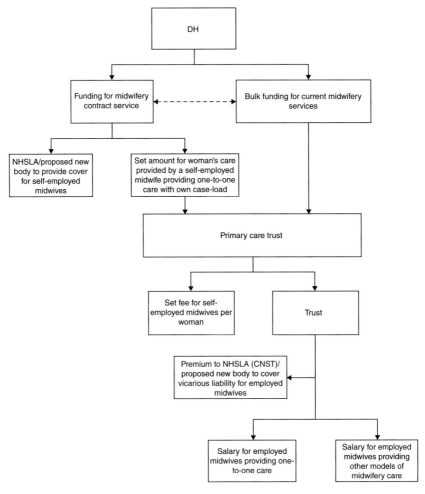

Figure 1.1 Funding the NHS Community Midwifery Model. (Reproduced with permission from *The Practising Midwife*, **9**, 23.) CNST, Clinical Negligence Scheme for Trusts.

Press releases report positive meetings with health ministers and key stakeholders concerning the proposed NHSCMM. It is still early days for the model and the next logical step would be the implementation of pilot projects. Anecdotally, there are some midwives in strategic posts who are suggesting wholesale change without this precursor. There have been numerous pilots since Caroline Flint first introduced the concept of team midwifery in the mid-1980s and we know that continuity of carer improves outcomes for mothers and babies. Women would clearly benefit if wholesale adoption of the OMOM campaign is realised. They would be able to choose a midwife who can support them throughout the duration of the childbearing experience, with all the benefits that continuity of carer brings. Access to NHS services and premises would be maintained, as would the existing traditional models of maternity care. The great advantage for midwives would be the potential to move between case-loading or hospital-based practice at particular times to suit their lifestyle demands and philosophies. The OMOM model does not, however, currently identify any proposed provision for midwives to move seamlessly between employment by the NHS and PCTs in relation to terms and conditions or pension rights (Figure 1.2).

The OMOM model could add an extra dimension to the four national choice guarantees proposed for 2009 (DH/PCFM, 2007) by extending the choice of carer. Overall, the proposal prompts consideration of the successful implementation of a similar system in New Zealand, where approximately 50% of practising midwives are now self-employed, with the remainder employed by district health boards (New Zealand College of Midwives, 2004).

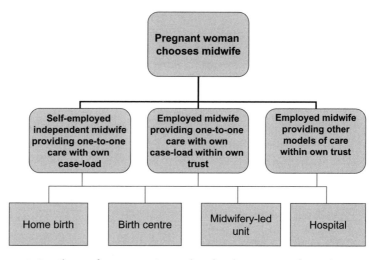

Figure 1.2 Choices for women. (Reproduced with permission from *The Practising Midwife*, **9**, 22.)

Primary healthcare trusts and practice-based commissioning

Should the NHSCMM or similar initiatives become a reality in the UK, individual midwives would effectively be able to contract out their services to PCTs. First established in 1997, PCTs now commission community, primary and secondary services for defined populations and are funded directly through budgets allocated by the DH. Talbot-Smith and Pollock (2006) indicate that the number of PCTs is being streamlined and that the envisaged proportion of PCTs to population is 1 : 500 000.

Each PCT is structured with two levels. The trust board is always made up of a majority of non-executive lay members who live locally and have experience of working at board level. The board works closely with the professional executive committee (PEC), which comprises clinicians from a wide range of professions. The PEC considers local needs, formulates proposals for the development of services and then presents those proposals for consideration by the board. It is relatively simple to discover the composition of any trust board or PEC in England via the web pages at: www.nhs,uk/England/AuthoritiesTrusts.

Midwives are not generally represented on PCTs because non-executive members of the board cannot be employees of the NHS. It is also a pre-requisite for members of a PEC to be employees of the relevant PCT.

The commissioning process is undertaken in partnership with other PCTs, GP practices and local authorities, and accountability is due directly to strategic health authorities (DH, 2006). One of the main advantages of the new commissioning system is the option for PCTs and practice-based commissioners to directly employ a range of professionals in order to expand the availability of local services within medical centres. The practice-based commissioning system offers scope to fund total packages of care but requires reform if midwives are to become truly involved in the process (Appleby, 2006). There are real opportunities for innovative managers and midwives but the current commissioning system does not facilitate midwifery involvement. Appleby identifies that devolved decision-making and the driver of the NSF will support the premise that primary care based models offer significant benefits for women and their babies. She then urges midwives to '. . . take up the mantle of modernisation. If we do not, then others who are not midwives will do it for us.'

Key considerations and initiatives

This introductory chapter has considered the potential to embrace new ways of working in the community. It would be impossible to detail every initiative forging ahead as a result of recent government reports, but three more topics will be highlighted in the following section: the development of children's centres, the Common Assessment Framework (CAF) and the role of maternity support workers. These have been chosen as key issues that community midwives will almost certainly be engaging with in the near future.

Children's centres

Jewell (2005) states that 'Sure Start is a shining example' of a multidisciplinary model that meets the needs of a community. The overall aim of Sure Start has been to address inequalities in health in targeted postcode areas across the UK and midwives have been working closely with other agencies to make it a success. Khazaezadeh (2005) describes how a small team of midwives implemented a case-loading approach to provide 'enhanced midwifery services to women from vulnerable and disadvantaged groups' in a Sure Start area, whilst simultaneously addressing public health targets such as improving breastfeeding rates and reducing smoking. She emphasises the need to adapt working practices to meet women's needs in identifying the value of 'drop in' services, outreach work and the provision of venues where women can meet together to establish social support networks.

The Sure Start initiative has been evaluated extensively over a period of 6 years. It is possible to read local evaluations from the extensive database compiled on the Birbeck, University of London (2007) *National Evaluation of Sure Start* pages. Local authorities have now been given strategic responsibility to build upon the work done by Sure Start to date through the development of children's centres. Centres will still be located in the most disadvantaged wards, with the remit of targeting services for potentially 650000 pre-school children (Department for Education and Skills, 2007). Every community should be served by a children's centre by 2010 (DH/PCFM, 2007) and services should evolve to meet specific local needs through extensive consultation with users. O'Sullivan (2005) suggests the possibility of further evolution through the creation of children's trusts, which could encompass maternity services to directly employ midwives in the future.

The Common Assessment Framework and multidisciplinary working

The development of children's centres has been heavily influenced by the green paper *Every Child Matters* (Department for Education and Skills, 2003). This document arose chiefly from Lord Laming's (2003) enquiry into the case of Victoria Climbié, which identified the tragic consequences when agencies fail to share key information effectively.

The close proximity of a number of agencies located within children's centres will facilitate multidisciplinary working to a great extent.

Professional groups have traditionally 'owned' their individual systems for collecting, storing and retrieving information, and this factor has precluded effective inter-agency information sharing to some degree. This has resulted in the need for clients from all walks of life, in need of support from a range of services, to regurgitate their histories and express their needs repeatedly as they engage with each organisation or professional group involved in their care. It is relatively easy to understand how this factor might have deterred vulnerable people from seeking support in the past.

Nationwide implementation of the CAF should be complete by 2008 (Department for Education and Skills, 2006a). The CAF is a standardised assessment tool that aims to identify the needs of a child or young adult in order to offer support and appropriate interventions as early as possible. It is very relevant for midwifery practice:

> 'The Common Assessment Framework can be used for children and young people of any age, including unborn babies' Department for Education and Skills (2006a)

The availability of the CAF can be viewed as reassuring. It is a tool that will support decision-making for community midwives, who often face dilemmas when caring for women who have complex needs or a lifestyle that potentially poses threats to a baby's health and well-being. Midwives aim to foster trust and confidence within their professional relationships with women. They can therefore experience a significant degree of anxiety when an instinctive need to gain a woman's trust conflicts with the statutory requirement to instigate a referral to protect the interests of babies and also their older siblings. The CAF is supported by clear guidance for professionals regarding the appropriate sharing of information and need for disclosure, with or without the client's consent (Department for Education and Skills, 2006b). Key advice urges the desirability of obtaining consent for disclosure through open, honest and early exchange of information with women, outlining the circumstances where disclosure is a professional and statutory requirement.

Case study 1.1 illustrates effective use of this tool.

Case study 1.1 Assessing the needs of the unborn child

Background
Telford & Wrekin and Shropshire is testing ways of working to improve information sharing amongst practitioners working with children. They have developed a working model focussed on early intervention, using common assessment to bring together a 'team around a child' to provide early support. Selbie, a senior midwife, provides a case study that illustrates how the programme has improved the delivery of children's services.

Early intervention

Susan was referred to Selbie when she was 12 weeks' pregnant. Selbie was concerned that Susan's learning difficulties may contribute to a need for extra support in fulfilling a parenting role. After the consultation, Selbie contacted her local information sharing and assessment coordinator to discuss her concern, and it was agreed that it would be helpful to complete a common assessment to define Susan's needs and work out a solution. They also agreed that early intervention was necessary to ensure Susan was ready to cope with the demands of parenthood, and that the well-being of the child, even the unborn child, must drive decisions.

Common assessment process

Selbie met with Susan and her mother, explained the assessment process and sought consent to share the assessment information with other practitioners. The completion of the common assessment meant that all Susan's needs were identified at an early stage, she did not have to repeat information to different agencies and she had ongoing support. The assessment process highlighted Susan's complex needs and as a result a team of practitioners, including a community midwife, social worker, health visitor, GP, Sure Start and community parenting worker, was formed to develop a plan to address Susan's needs.

Lead professional

It was agreed that the health visitor should assume the role of lead professional as her involvement with the family would be ongoing. Support was provided for Susan to attend appropriate antenatal care and to provide one-to-one support to help her develop her parenting skills. The health visitor provided a link with Susan and the other professionals, both during her pregnancy and in the early stages of parenthood.

Outcome

The support network offered helped Susan understand the need to look after her unborn child and facilitated the development of her parenting skills. She has the continued support of her health worker, with whom she has built trust and can call on if she needs further help with her child.

(Department for Education and Skills, 2006c)

The lead professional role primarily addresses the co-ordination of services to ensure consistency and is often identified following a multi-agency review generated by the CAF. The designated lead professional may change as the client's needs evolve. Families with complex needs will make contact with numerous professional groups, and local systems are being developed to enable practitioners to access common assessments and update them as necessary.

The simplest way for community midwives to find out whether a CAF has already been completed is to ask the woman herself.

A national information sharing index known as Contact Point should be available from 2008 to ensure that children who move from area to area, or who access services across traditional boundaries, are not lost to the system. Contact Point will contain baseline information such as the name, address, gender and date of birth of a child and related contact details for relevant agencies. Access to the index will be restricted but all health professionals will be able to seek advice and information via a designated local contact or lead professional.

Maternity support workers

The NHS Employers National Large-Scale Workforce Change (LSWC) team is part of the NHS confederation. In 2005 they led a 10-month programme, involving 55 NHS trusts, to implement the maternity support worker (MSW) role. A two-fold rationale for the programme is clearly stated in the resulting report: to support the implementation of Standard 11 of the NSF and to improve the working lives of practising midwives (NHS Employers, 2006). The aims of the programme are:

- to develop and implement MSW roles as an integrated part of the team in ante- and postnatal periods across hospital and community care settings
- to reduce midwifery time spent on non-clinical tasks
- to address the retention and recruitment issues of midwives and other related staff
- to assist in the development of a career/education framework for MSWs
- to improve the working lives of staff delivering maternity services
- to support compliance with the European Working Time Directive by 2009.

(NHS Employers, 2006: 4)

The LSWC team supported project leads and teams within each participating trust, sharing their expertise in the management of workforce change. Core outcomes reported upon were the number of MSW posts implemented and the amount of midwifery time released as a result. Trust teams were then asked to identify how this newly available midwifery time was being used to improve the quality of service provision. The programme mapped the introduction of 218 whole-time equivalent posts and the report presents a positive evaluation of the initiative from service users, midwives and the MSWs themselves.

Sandall et al. (2007) have recently presented the results of a national scoping study of the implementation of the MSW role in NHS trusts in England. Feedback obtained from managers indicates that they generally view the role as a positive one, but a number of issues for concern are identified. These include a wide variation in the nature of the skills and tasks that are being delegated to MSWs, and Sandall et al. (2007) highlight an urgent need to clarify the boundaries in order to protect both the public and the midwifery profession. They also suggest that it may not be appropriate for MSWs to take on new competencies and that consideration should be given instead to employing a greater number of MSWs in their traditional supporting role. Most worryingly, and in direct contrast to the NHS Employers (2006) stated aim to improve recruitment and retention of midwives, 51% of the units responding to the scoping exercise indicated that they are addressing midwifery vacancy gaps through conversion of midwifery posts to MSW posts.

Implementation of the role of the MSW across all care settings prompts examination of relevant advice to clarify the related responsibilities of the midwife. MSWs will increasingly play a part in meeting the needs of the maternity services as part of the workforce planning strategy so it is crucial that midwives are clear about the boundaries of the role.

The Nursing and Midwifery Council (NMC) update relating to delegation of care states clearly that midwives are professionally accountable for any care task delegated to an unregistered healthcare support worker (NMC, 2006).

If the support worker has been trained and assessed as competent by their employer, the worker then assumes responsibility for the care given and this should be reflected in the individual's contract of employment, to include vicarious liability. In the event that a midwife considers that a support worker does not have a particular competency, or that delegation is inappropriate, she/he can decline a request to delegate care. The Code of Professional Conduct supports this action (NMC, 2004) and the NMC advises that a midwife should raise any issues arising with their employer, in writing.

The LSWC project (NHS Employers, 2006) is set within an overall imperative for the NHS to plan services for the future. Unregulated support workers have already been aligned to many services inside and outside the NHS. Teachers are working with classroom assistants, the police force are working with community support officers and midwives will increasingly be working with MSWs in the future. A team approach towards provision of care is clearly part of the plan.

Critique of the National Service Framework

The assertion that midwives must expand their role to meet the expectations of the NSF has been questioned by Robinson (2004a), who expresses concern about the current poor levels of midwifery staffing. This stance may readily and understandably be echoed by many practitioners, but it can be challenged. Community midwives, in particular, have always been engaged in promoting the health of the population in general, but that work has been implicit and not readily acknowledged. The NSF aims to promote a more explicit public health related role for midwives, through supporting new initiatives and best practice.

There are many examples to indicate that community midwifery practice is evolving already (DH, 2003) and traditional ways of working in the community are being questioned. One as yet under-reported example concerns the way that women access postnatal care. Home visits are being minimised in some areas through the option for women to meet their midwives by appointment at designated locations in the community and this concept has been adopted as a national choice guarantee (DH/PCFM, 2007). As maternity services are re-energised and reorganised around a range of initiatives, in response to the needs of the community, it is feasible to suggest that midwifery recruitment and retention rates can improve.

Robinson (2004b) continues to identify that the NSF echoes many of the key messages of *Changing Childbirth* to intimate that it might be foolhardy to expect a great deal from the NSF when its precursor failed to deliver significant improvements. This view is countered by many (Richens and Thomas, 2004; Dimond, 2005; Gould et al., 2005) who emphasise the fact that there is a mandatory element compelling NHS trusts to respond to the NSF. This manifests as statutory provision for independent bodies to audit the quality of maternity services against the benchmark of Standard 11. This process aims to establish minimum levels of service, which can then be built upon as external scrutiny continues, thus eliminating local variations in service provision.

One very difficult question remains: How do Standard 11 of the NSF and *Maternity Matters* fit in with the increasing centralisation of maternity services? Bones' (2005) critique of centralisation highlights the overriding economic basis underpinning the closure of many popular midwife-led community units. She cites a number of negative consequences for women, including diminished choice for the place of birth and the perpetuation of a medically dominated model of care. There is a degree of conflict between the goals of the NSF and *Maternity Matters* to deliver a range of individualised and accessible local maternity services, and the wider financial remit for NHS trusts to balance their books. Ratnaike (2007) points out that the Royal College of Midwives has calculated that 3000 more whole-time equivalent midwifery posts are needed to meet the DH's proposals in full. The potential for the development of community-based initiatives on a large scale could be subsumed in the future by the needs of the organisation as a whole.

Summary

This chapter has reviewed events which have shaped the role of the community midwife in the past, and some of the factors that will determine it in the 21st century. The context of childbearing and the ways in which community midwives work have clearly been subject to the influence of government reports over time. The NHS 10-year plan augurs further change as it continues to unfold. Future plans indicate a clear focus upon the midwife's role within the wider public health agenda and a professed desire to meet the majority of low-risk childbearing women's needs through community-based services. The DH and associated agencies have produced a wealth of documentation to guide practitioners. Key documents relating to the role of the community midwife have been highlighted and it is hoped that these pointers will prompt practitioners to explore some of them in greater depth.

There is also a heightened expectation, driven by clinical governance, for community midwives to consistently provide high quality, evidence-based care. Services will be mapped alongside and measured against the standards laid out by the NSF. Richens and Thomas (2004) state that it is time to make a cultural shift – to move away from a traditionally focused mindset that prioritises the organisation, towards services designed to meet the local needs of women and their families. Gould et al. (2005) talk about 'inverting the hierarchy' to achieve this goal but they also remind us of Kirkham's (2000) assertion that 'midwives would often support the system rather than deliver individualised care'. The need for strong leadership is clear.

The remaining chapters of this book will address selected topics pertinent to the role of the midwife based in the community. The information offered aims to go some way towards supporting those midwives in their goal to achieve excellence in all they do for women and their families.

Reflection postscript

More than 7 years after leaving the community to work in a consultant unit labour ward, I bumped into one of the traveller women's husbands as he waited outside the unit for news of the birth of his grandchild. Staff had expressed reservations about a fierce-looking character that had been pacing the corridor – and I have to agree that he does indeed have a striking demeanour.

To my joy he greeted me as a long-lost friend. We caught up on family news and I was reminded, once again, why my time in the community was so valuable. Without that experience it is highly likely that I would have fallen in line with my consultant unit colleagues and approached the man very differently.

> ⚷ **Key points**
>
> - Community midwives have real opportunities to engage with women and their families over a period of time.
> - Community midwives have always been engaged with public health work.
> - Expansion of the community midwife's role in public health is dependent upon multidisciplinary working and the appropriate implementation of the MSW role.
> - The NSF for Maternity Services and the *Maternity Matters* report are supportive of new initiatives, such as case-loading, that meet local needs – but there is a pressing need to increase the number of practising midwives to meet the proposed agenda.
> - Strong leadership is vital to ensure midwifery representation and involvement in the practice-based commissioning process.

References

Appleby, S. (2006) Engaging with the challenge of change. *Midwives*, **9** (8), 302–305.

Ball, L., Curtis, P. and Kirkham, M. (2002) *Why do Midwives Leave?* Royal College of Midwives, London.

Barber, T. (1998) Stress and the management of change. *Midwives Journal*, **1**, 26–27.

Birbeck, University of London (2007) National Evaluation of Sure Start – Local Evaluation Findings. www.ness.bbk.ac.uk/findings.asp (accessed 26.2.07).

Bones, E. (2005) The true cost of the centralization of maternity services. *MIDIRS*, **15** (4), 559–564.

Campbell, R. and Macfarlane, A. (1994) *Where to be Born? The Debate and the Evidence*. National Perinatal Epidemiology Unit, Oxford.

Curtis, P., Ball, L. and Kirkham, M. (2006) Working together? Indices of division in the midwifery workforce. *British Journal of Midwifery*, **14** (3), 138–141.

Declercq, E. (1998) Changing Childbirth in the United Kingdom: Lessons for US Health Policy. *Journal of Health Politics, Policy & Law*, **23** (5), 833–850.

Department for Education and Skills (2003) *Every Child Matters*. The Stationery Office, London.

Department for Education and Skills (2006a) *Making it happen: Working together for children, young people and families*. Department for Education and Skills, London.

Department for Education and Skills (2006b) *The Common Assessment Framework for Children and Young People: Supporting Tools. Integrated Working to Improve Outcomes for Children and Young People*. Department for Education and Skills, London.

Department for Education and Skills (2006c) *The Common Assessment Framework for Children & Young People: Supporting Tools. Integrated Working to Improve Outcomes for Children and Young People.* (Crown Copyright applies – ref: Alex Clabburn), Department for Education and Skills, London.

Department for Education and Skills (2007) Children's Centres. www. standards.dfes.gov.uk/primary/faqs/foundation_stage/1162267/ #1162271 (accessed 26.2.07).

DH (1993) *Changing Childbirth: The Report of the Expert Maternity Group.* HMSO, London.

DH (1998) *A First Class Service: Quality in the New NHS.* The Stationery Office, London.

DH (2000) *The NHS Plan: A Plan for Investment, a Plan for Reform.* The Stationery Office, London.

DH (2003) *Delivering the Best: Midwives Contribution to the NHS Plan.* The Stationery Office, London.

DH (2004) *National Service Framework for Children, Young People and Maternity Services: Maternity services.* Department of Health/Department for Education and Skills, London.

DH (2006) PCT and SHA roles and functions. www.dh.gov.uk (accessed 22/11/06).

DH/PCFM (2007) *Maternity Matters: Choice, Access and Continuity of Care in a Safe Service.* Department of Health/Partnerships for Children, Families and Maternity, London.

Dimond, B. (2005) Will the NSF be more successful than Cumberledge? *British Journal of Midwifery*, **13** (2), 106.

Flint, C. (1986) The Know Your Midwife Scheme. *Midwife, Health Visitor and Community Nurse*, **22**, 168–169.

Francis, A. and van der Kooy, B. (2004) 21st-century midwifery: NHS community midwifery models. *AIMS Journal*, **16** (2), 2004.

Gould, D., Hogarth, S. and Stephens, L. (2005) Inverting the hierarchy. *Midwives*, **8** (8), 354–355.

Hart, A. and Lockey, R. (2002) Inequalities in healthcare provision: the relationship between contemporary policy and contemporary practice in maternity services in England. *Journal of Advanced Nursing*, **37** (5), 485–493.

Hicks, C., Spurgeon, P. and Barwell, F. (2003) Changing Childbirth: a pilot project. *Journal of Advanced Nursing*, **42** (6), 617–628.

Hindley, J. (2005) Having a baby in Balsall Heath: women's experiences and views of continuity and discontinuity of midwifery care in the mother–midwife relationship. *MIDIRS Midwifery Digest*, **15** (4), S35-47, Supplement 2.

Hodnett, E.D. (2004) Continuity of caregivers for care during pregnancy and childbirth (Cochrane review). *The Cochrane Library*, Issue 2.

Hunter, B. (2004) Conflicting ideologies as a source of emotion work in midwifery. *Midwifery*, **20**, 261–272.

Jewell, K. (2005) The public health divide. *Midwives*, **8** (7), 318–319.

Khan, I. and Pillay, K. (2003) Users' attitudes towards home and hospital treatment: a comparative study between South Asian and white residents of the British Isles. *Journal of Psychiatric & Mental Health Nursing*, **10** (2),137–146.

Khazaezadeh, N. (2005) Benefits of Sure Start caseload midwifery. *Midwives*, **8** (10), 422–423.

Kirkham, M. (2000) *The Midwife–Mother Relationship.* Palgrave Macmillan, Basingstoke.

Lewis, G. (ed) (2001) *Why Mothers Die 1997–1999 – Report on Confidential Enquiries into Maternal Deaths in the United Kingdom.* RCOG, London.

Lewis, G. (ed) (2004) *Why Mothers Die 2000–2002 – Report on Confidential Enquiries into Maternal Deaths in the United Kingdom.* RCOG, London.

Lord Laming (2003) *The Victoria Climbié Inquiry.* The Stationery Office, London.

Ministry of Health (1959) *Report of the Maternity Services Committee (Chairman, Lord Cranbrook).* HMSO, London.

Munro, A. (chair) (1984) *Maternity Care in Action Part 2: Care During Childbirth. Second Report of the Maternity Services Advisory Committee to the Secretaries of State for Social Services and for Wales.* HMSO, London.

New Zealand College of Midwives (2004) *Midwifery Practice in New Zealand.* New Zealand College of Midwives. www.midwife.org.nz/index.cfm/ Practice (accessed 26.2.07).

NHS Employers (2006) Maternity Support Workers: Enhancing the Work of the Maternity Team. www.nhsemployers.org (accessed 12.9.07).

NMC (2004) *The NMC Code of Professional Conduct: Standards for Conduct, Performance and Ethics.* Nursing and Midwifery Council, London.

NMC (2006) Delegation of Care Update. October, Nursing and Midwifery Council, London. www.nmc-uk.org (accessed 28.2.07).

O'Sullivan, S. (2005) Health care outside of hospital. In: *News and Appointments: Mid-month Supplement.* Royal College of Midwives, October, p. 4.

Ratnaike, D. (2007) Is choice the answer? *Midwives*, **10** (6), 264.

Reid, B. (2002a) The Albany Midwifery Practice. *MIDIRS Midwifery Digest*, **14** (1), 118–121.

Reid, B. (2002b) The Albany Midwifery Practice (2). *MIDIRS Midwifery Digest*, **12** (2), 261–264.

Richens, Y. and Thomas, M. (2004) Service framework calls for cultural shift. *British Journal of Midwifery*, **12** (11), 668–670.

Robinson, J. (2004a) Prolonged midwifery care: where will we find the midwives? *British Journal of Midwifery*, **12** (10), 642.

Robinson, J. (2004b) Sweet and sour – the National Service Framework. *British Journal of Midwifery*, **12** (11), 892.

Rosser, J. (2003) How do the Albany Midwives do it? Evaluation of the Albany Midwives Practice. *MIDIRS Midwifery Digest*, **1** (2), 251–257.

Sandall, J. (1997) Midwives' burnout and continuity of care. *British Journal of Midwifery*, **5** (2), 106–111.

Sandall, J., Davies, J. and Warwick, C. (2001) *Evaluation of the Albany Midwifery Practice: Final Report*. Florence Nightingale School of Nursing and Midwifery, Kings College London, London.

Sandall, J., Manthorpe, J., Mansfield, A. and Spencer, L. (2007) *Support Workers in Maternity Services: a national scoping study of NHS Trusts providing maternity care in England 2006. Final Report*. Kings College London, London.

Standing Maternity and Midwifery Advisory Committee (Chairman, J. Peel) (1970). *Domiciliary Midwifery and Maternity Bed Needs*. HMSO, London.

Talbot, S.A. and Pollock, A. (2006) *The New NHS: A Guide*. Routledge, London.

Tinkler, A. and Quinney, D. (1998) Team midwifery: the influence of the midwife–woman relationship on women's experiences and perceptions of maternity care. *Journal of Advanced Nursing*, **28** (1), 30–35.

Wraight, A., Ball, J., Secombe, I. and Stock, J. (1993) *Mapping Team Midwifery*. Institute of Manpower Studies, University of Sussex, Brighton.

Birth

Watching and waiting: the facilitation of birth at home

Kim Russell

'The midwife herself shall sit before the labouring woman . . . offer sweet words, giving her hope of a good speed in deliverance.' Rayhald (1545)

Normal birth has been defined as a vaginal birth without instruments, induction, epidural or general anaesthetic (DH, 2005; BirthChoiceUK, 2006). Using this definition, the number of vaginal births has fallen nationally from 65% in 1990 to 46% in 2004. The number of normal births supported by midwives is falling because of the increase in caesarean sections and the use of epidural anaesthesia (Office of National Statistics, 2004; DH, 2005).

In 2002, 96% of births in the UK took place in hospital units (Office of National Statistics, 2004). Davis-Floyd (1992) states that we have to recognise that medical intervention in normal labour may be acceptable and even welcomed by some women, but many have expressed a lack of satisfaction with hospitals when compared with home or birth centre care (Walsh, 2002; Kirkham, 2003). Since the publication of *Changing Childbirth* (DH, 1993), the concept of women's choice and control over options for maternity care has become widely accepted in society, but it could be argued that the high rate of hospital birth does not reflect individual choice. It could indicate that the current system encourages conformity and places limits on women's options for the place of birth.

Over the last century, many countries in the western world have organised maternity services around a medical model of care where childbirth takes place in hospital (Wagner, 1995; Davis-Floyd and Sargent, 1997; DeVries and Barroso, 1997; Tew, 1998; Kirkham, 2000; Kitzinger, 2005). The medicalisation of birth has been likened to an industrial production line where women are viewed as machines and babies as products, to be processed as quickly as possible (Davis-Floyd, 1992; Perkins, 2004).

Perkins (2004) describes how systems of care, within the NHS, have adopted management models which value efficiency and effectiveness. This has led to small units and birth centres throughout the UK being closed and women's choice in place of birth being reduced. However, the need to increase home births for women with low-risk pregnancies has been recognised in both the National Service Framework for maternity care (DH, 2004) and the *Maternity Matters* report (DH/PCFM, 2007).

A study undertaken by the National Childbirth Trust (NCT) found that 22% of women in the UK would like to give birth at home (Singh and Newburn, 2000), but despite this finding home births currently account for just 2.14% of all UK births (BirthChoiceUK, 2006). A geographical variation exists and between regions this ranges from less than 1% to over 20% (RCM, 2002). The reasons for this geographical variation may be due to the negative or positive attitudes of healthcare professionals towards home birth and how maternity systems are organised. The negative attitudes of many doctors are well-documented (NCT, 2001), but Hosein (1998) found that midwives' personal beliefs also acted as a barrier to women being offered choice about place of birth. In reality, it appears that many midwives select women they think are suitable for home birth rather than offering true choice (Floyd, 1995; Anderson, 2002). Walsh (2000) believes that there is an inherent bias against home birth within the current system, which results in women not being offered this option.

Evidence-based practice

It was thought that the introduction of evidence-based practice would facilitate client choice as it encourages active participation in the decision-making process (Cluett and Bluff, 2000; Sackett et al., 2002). This chapter identifies the principles of evidence-based midwifery and how midwives can apply these principles in clinical practice. Evidence-based midwifery care is based on the principles set out in *Changing Childbirth* (DH, 1993), *Effective Care in Pregnancy and Childbirth* (Enkin et al., 2000) and evidence-based medicine. The use of evidence-based practice aims to increase practitioners' knowledge by utilising research skills and reflective practice to enhance clinical decision-making (Sackett et al., 2002). The following stages offer a framework that can be worked through to ensure that midwives are practising evidence-based midwifery:

Step 1: Find out what is important to the woman and her family
Step 2: Use information from clinical assessment
Step 3: Seek and appraise evidence to inform decision-making

Step 4: Talk it through and reflect on possible outcomes and feelings (Adapted from Page, 2000: 10)

Case study 2.1 demonstrates how these stages of evidence-based practice might be used by community midwives. It is based on a true case but the names and places have been changed to ensure confidentiality (NMC, 2004a).

Case study 2.1 Meeting Andrea

I met Andrea for the first time at her home, to carry out a 12-week booking interview. She had recently moved to the area so we had not met before. During the booking interview Andrea told me that she was expecting her second child. Her daughter, Phoebe, was now 3 years old. Phoebe had been born at a consultant unit hospital without any complications. Andrea found her first labour quite daunting but felt she coped well with the contractions, using 'gas and air' and pethidine during her 12-hour labour. Andrea and her husband Dave were quite happy with their previous experience and were content to have this baby in another consultant-led maternity unit.

Step 1: Find out what is important to the woman and her family

Assessing what was important to Andrea and her family was difficult at our first meeting, but from what she said it was clear that Andrea's previous birth was a positive experience. Some midwives may feel that given Andrea's satisfaction with hospital birth there was no need to discuss home birth as an option, but it could be argued that, unless the place of birth is discussed, Andrea and Dave are not making an informed choice. Some women may not reach a decision on home birth until the end of pregnancy. By this point, the prospect of labour is very real to both the woman and her partner, and a trusting relationship between the mother and midwife has been established. The Albany Practice midwives ask women from their case-load where they would like to give birth once their labours have started. At this time the woman is more able to choose the safest place for herself and her baby. This approach has resulted in a 45% home birth rate (Albany Midwifery Practice, 2003).

Step 2: Use information from clinical assessment

During the booking interview, it is usual to take a full medical and family history to identify any possible risk factors and it is also important to explore the woman's psychological and social history in order to offer

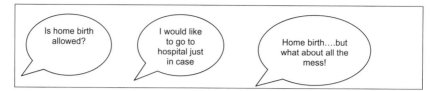

Figure 2.1   Common responses from women and their partners.

appropriate care and advice (Page, 2000). I undertook a detailed obstetric history and a full physical examination in order to make an accurate assessment of Andrea's risk of pregnancy or labour complications. Assessment of risk has become an important aspect of the community midwife's role and a central part of risk management approaches (Johnson, 2000).

Andrea was assessed as low risk because of her previous normal birth history and lack of medical or social risk factors. Olsen and Jewell (2002) recommend that all women with low-risk pregnancies should be offered the opportunity of having their babies at home.

When you first discuss having a baby at home, women and their partners are often surprised or even shocked. They respond in a variety of ways (Figure 2.1).

Women and their partners are often concerned about the safety of home birth because they believe that home is a dangerous place to have a baby and hospital is the safest option (Stephens, 2005). In medical models of care, safety is seen as an absolute concept focused on mortality and morbidity (Woodcock et al., 1994; Tew, 1998). In relation to maternal death, giving birth has never been safer but over recent decades the concept of risk has changed to demonstrate an increasing focus on the fetus (Queniart, 1992).

According to the DH (2004), 'all women should be involved in planning their own care with information, advice and support from professionals' but women often choose to give birth in hospital because, like their mothers before them, they perceive it to be the safest place (Allison, 1996). This perception may also be due to fears about the pain of labour and birth and the desire to have access to pain-relieving drugs (Green et al., 1998). Anderson (2002: 12) argues that the way to reduce young women's fears of birth is to increase the number of home births so that women 'see birth as something not to fear'. By encouraging birth at home, midwives can offer an opportunity for younger women to observe and learn about normal childbirth. This may go some way towards changing perceptions and informing future choices.

Step 3: Seek and appraise evidence to inform decision-making

In Andrea and Dave's case their concerns were centred on the safety of home birth. My role was to help Andrea make an informed choice about the place of birth by providing her with current research evidence as well as information about the benefits and risks of hospital birth (Davis, 2004). It was also important to provide information about induction rates, infection rates and birth outcomes of the local hospital obstetric unit. Leaflets such as the *MIDIRS Midwifery Digest* informed choice leaflets and websites such as the Association for Improvements in Maternity Care (AIMS, 2006) may also be helpful.

Women and their partners differ in the amount of detail they require to make informed decisions. Some may try and find their own evidence whereas others will be quite happy to make decisions based on the information provided by their midwife. In either case, the woman and her partner should be given ample opportunity to ask questions and seek clarification on the information provided so that an informed choice about where to give birth can be reached.

Is home birth safe?

The safety of home birth has been debated for decades. It is apparent that popular culture in the UK believes birth at home to be more dangerous than hospital birth but there is currently no evidence to support this assumption (RCM, 2002). Anderson (2002) argues convincingly that the biggest intervention in the birth process is asking women to leave their place of safety to give birth in hospital, and current research indicates that home birth is a safe option for women experiencing low-risk pregnancies. Studies carried out over the last 10 years demonstrate quite clearly that women who plan to give birth at home are more likely to give birth vaginally (see Table 2.1).

The recent draft intrapartum guidelines devised by the National Institute for Clinical Excellence (NICE, 2006) recognise that birth outside consultant-led units improves outcomes for women. However, NICE have questioned the outcomes for babies born at home because of the apparent variation in perinatal mortality rates (PMR) in the studies they reviewed. They have recommended that further research is needed before any conclusions about the safety of home birth for babies can be reached. Until further research evidence becomes available midwives, other professionals and parents have the clear option to refer to existing studies that have shown neonatal outcomes at home are no worse than hospital birth for women with low-risk pregnancies (Olsen and Jewell, 2002). The recent draft intrapartum guidelines also recognise that birth outside hospital is associated with higher levels of maternal satisfaction (NICE, 2006).

It might be helpful here to consider the wider benefits of home birth for Andrea and her family.

Table 2.1 Summary of key research evidence.

Research	Methods	Findings	Conclusions
Northern Region Perinatal Mortality Survey Coordinating Group (1996) Collaborative survey of perinatal loss in planned and unplanned homebirths. *BMJ*, **313** (Nov), 1306–1309	Survey of 558 691 births over a 13-year period	Perinatal problems mainly unavoidable in planned homebirth group	Poor perinatal outcomes much less common in the homebirth group
Doweswell, T., Thornton, J., Hewison, J., Lilford, R. (1996) Should there be a trial of home versus hospital delivery in the United Kingdom? *BMJ*, **312**, 753–757	Small randomised control trial of 11 women	No differences in outcomes between home and hospital deliveries were found apart from disappointment in the hospital group as to their allocation	No differences between hospital and home birth outcomes
Chamberlain, G., Wraight, A., Cowley, P. (1997) *Home Births: The Report of the Confidential Enquiry by the National Birthday Trust Fund.* Carnforth Partheon Publishing Group	Randomised control trial 6000 women who planned a home birth at 37 weeks matched with women who planned a hospital birth	Higher rates of instrumental and caesarean section rates in hospital group Women at home had lower rates of episiotomies, PPH and used less pharmacological analgesia Babies born at home had higher apgar scores	Women who have normal pregnancies prior to home birth are at no greater risk than a woman who gives birth in hospital
Tew, M. (1998) *Safer Childbirth. A Critical History of Maternity Care*	Retrospective analysis	The PMR for planned home birth were better than in hospital	Babies born at a planned home birth had better PMR than in hospital

Reference	Method	Findings	Conclusions
RCOG (1998) CESDI-5th Annual Report. RCOG Press, London	Reviewed 22 home births which resulted in the death of a baby. Included women and babies transferred to hospital	Sub-optimal care was identified in the home birth group – the same issues in deaths that occurred in hospital were identified	Sub-optimal care was NO more likely to occur at home
Olsen, O., Jewell, M.D. (2002) Home versus hospital birth (Cochrane Review): In: The Cochrane Library, issue 1. Update Software, Oxford	Meta analysis. The main objective was to review the effects of planned home birth compared to hospital rates of interventions, complications and morbidity	The rates of dystocia, fetal distress, low apgars, neonatal respiratory problems and birth trauma were higher for planned hospital births. The rates of excessive bleeding and retained placenta were lower in the planned hospital group	There is no strong evidence to favour either hospital birth or planned home birth for low-risk women. All low-risk pregnant women should be offered a planned home birth
NICE (2006) Draft intrapartum guideline. Consultation ends August 2006	Systematic literature review of current research evidence	Birth outside of consultant-led units is consistently associated with an increase in vaginal births, intact perineums and an increase in maternal satisfaction. Important variations in PMR difficult to quantify due to poor evidence	Urgently need further evidence that can quantify the benefit and risk of different birth settings. Recognised the need to investigate women's psychological/emotional well-being after birth

The psycho-social benefits of home birth

Higher levels of satisfaction have been reported by women who give birth at home compared with those who choose hospital, implying that medical systems of care often fail to meet women's psychological needs (Walsh, 2000a; Gibbons and Thomson, 2001). Birth is acknowledged as a significant event in a woman's life and the quality of the birth experience is important (Kitzinger, 2000). Research findings are increasingly telling us that a difficult birth can negatively affect the mother–baby relationship and women's levels of self-esteem (Fisher, 2002; Rowe-Murray and Fisher, 2002). Women who plan to give birth at home may have a more positive experience because they undoubtedly have higher levels of control over their own labours (Morison et al., 1998; Andrews, 2004; Box 2.1). Simkin (1992) has shown that this sense of control during childbirth may have positive benefits for the women concerned for 20 years or more. Feelings of empowerment also appear to help women cope better with the pain of labour (Edwards, 2005).

Box 2.1 Comments from women concerning control

'It was just so lovely and calm. The curtains were closed, it was a lovely day, we had a bit of music on. It was relaxed.'

'It's under your control, you call the shots. You phone the midwife when you want them.'

'Because I was in control I had a voice and you feel as if you can probably say to the midwife if you weren't happy.'

Andrews (2004: 552)

In addition to the issue of control, women are more likely to experience continuity of carer and continual support at home (Mander, 2001), both of which have been shown to improve birth outcomes (Hodnett et al., 2002). Kinsey (2005), a practising midwife, describes how the birth of her own child at home made her feel confident about her body's ability to give birth. She also touches on the social benefits of not having to leave her other child or the familiar surroundings of home.

Step 4: Talk it through and reflect on possible outcomes and feelings

After exploring the risks and benefits of hospital and home birth, Andrea and Dave decided to plan for the birth of their second child at home (Case study 2.2).

Case study 2.2 Andrea's home birth

I was called to Andrea's house at 7am on a sunny July morning. When I arrived, Andrea was contracting strongly and walking around the garden accompanied by her mother. Dave was giving Phoebe her breakfast. When I examined Andrea she was already 9 cm dilated. I called a second midwife to attend as Andrea's mother took over the care of Phoebe so that Dave could be by his wife's side. Baby Daniel was born onto his parents' bed 1 hour later. Daniel cried spontaneously and Andrea lifted him up into her arms to keep him warm.

The placenta and membranes were delivered with maternal effort and blood loss was minimal. Andrea and Dave were thrilled with their home birth!

In the past, health professionals have been recognised as being reluctant to provide women with information on which to make decisions (Mander, 2001). The use of the four-step process helps the midwife to put the woman and her family at the centre of the decision-making process, facilitating access to appropriate, evidence-based midwifery care. Use of this staged approach may also assist the development of a trusting midwife–mother relationship, recognised as central to the provision of effective midwifery care (Kirkham, 2000).

A right to home birth?

For many years there has been a perception that women have a legal right to have their baby at home with a trained midwife in attendance, but in 1995 NHS trusts realised that they had no legal obligation to provide a home birth service (AIMS, 2005). Conversely, it is also important to point out that no law exists to force a mentally competent woman to give birth in hospital (Lord Hunt of Kings Heath, 2000).

If an NHS trust withdraws its home birth service, it places community midwives in a difficult position: as an employed midwife you have a contractual duty to your employer. The Royal College of Midwives (RCM) produced a position paper which aimed to clarify the role and responsibilities of the midwives in relation to home birth (RCM, 2002). In reality, this kind of dilemma is rare but the RCM states that:

> 'It is good practice, and congruent with Government policy, to support women's informed choices and to promote home birth as a good option for women experiencing uncomplicated pregnancies.' RCM (2002)

Midwives have a contractual responsibility to their employer but also a professional duty to work within the Midwives Rules and Standards (NMC, 2004b) as well as the Code of Professional Conduct (NMC, 2004a). In August 2004 a community midwife, Paul Beland, was sacked after attending a woman in labour at a planned home birth. The

NHS trust concerned had withdrawn its home birth service because of staff shortages (BBC News, 2004). This case left many midwives confused about their legal and professional responsibilities. In 2006, the Nursing and Midwifery Council (NMC) issued further guidance:

> 'Should a conflict arise between service provision and a woman's choice for place of birth, a midwife has a duty of care to attend her. This is no different to a woman who has walked into a maternity unit to receive care.' NMC (2006b)

In essence, if such a conflict arises, the midwife concerned should communicate with her midwifery managers and supervisor of midwives to try and resolve the situation (Figure 2.2) (RCM, 2002; NMC, 2006b).

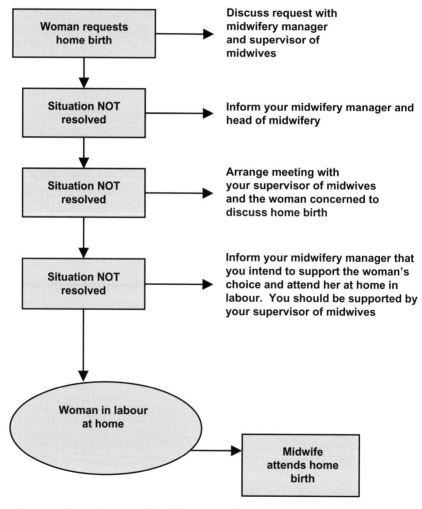

Figure 2.2 Resolving conflict of interests when an NHS trust withdraws its home birth service.

Remember that a supervisor of midwives has a duty to assist midwives in supporting women's choices (NMC, 2004b) and should be able to offer advice and support. Ultimately, if the situation cannot be resolved then the midwife should attend the home birth with the support of her supervisor of midwives. If the midwife has communicated fully with her employers and her supervisor of midwives, she or he will have endeavoured to meet both her contractual and professional duties.

The midwife, home birth and competence

The RCM (2002) recognises that home birth is central to the role of the midwife as the expert in normal birth and that midwifery support should be available as an integral part of maternity services. The NMC (2006b) states:

> 'Midwives are experts in normal birth, and the NMC standards require them to be competent to support women to give birth normally in a variety of settings, including the home.'

Unfortunately, because of the small numbers of home births in many parts of the UK, it may be difficult to ensure that midwives are competent in caring for women in non-medical environments. In fact, Anderson (2002) argues that most midwives are not specially trained for home birth. Stephens (2005) suggests creating designated home birth teams where expertise in home birth could be fostered. These teams would also be a valuable resource in training students and midwives. If you are starting your career as a community midwife with no local birth centres and a low home birth rate, however, how do you gain the experience you need? Box 2.2 offers some practical suggestions related to gaining experience and building the confidence you need to successfully facilitate birth at home.

Box 2.2 Suggested ways of gaining experience in home birth

Help yourself
Put yourself on call as a second midwife or ask to shadow an experienced midwife the next time a woman is planning a home birth. Talk to midwifery colleagues about their experiences. In this way you can learn about clinical decision making in the home and gain useful tips and insights.

Organise learning opportunities
Discuss the possibility of spending some time in a birth centre, midwifery group practice or with an independent midwife with your manager and supervisor of midwives. These visits could be used to meet your PREP requirements. In the unlikely event that your manger is unsupportive consider taking these opportunities for updating in your own time.

Continued

Policies
Make sure you have access to local policies and guidelines on home birth. In particular, make yourself familiar with the transfer procedures, equipment and drugs used in your local NHS trust. It is also important to read books and journals to support current best practice.

Emergencies
Practise your skills in all obstetric emergencies in a home situation. Make time to do this with fellow community midwives at regular intervals and always check the emergency equipment you carry routinely to ensure it is in good working order.

Physiology of labour and birth

To support women in giving birth at home effectively it is essential for midwives to have a clear understanding of normal birth physiology. Without this fundamental knowledge it is difficult to develop the appropriate skills that will facilitate physiological labour and birth. This section will identify key labour physiology and related traditional midwifery skills.

McNabb (1997) identifies the primary labour and birth hormones as oxytocin, beta-endorphin, the catecholamines (adrenaline and noradrenaline) and prolactin (Figure 2.3). It is important to note that physiological labour is supported by a 'complex yet delicate hormonal orchestration of labour and birth' (Buckley, 2004).

Most of the birth hormones identified are secreted from the primitive part of the brain known as the limbic system (McNabb, 1997). The levels of these hormones increase during physiological labour, reaching a peak at the time of birth (Buckley, 2004). In order for labour to progress physiologically, the limbic system needs to dominate the new brain (or neocortex) as this is responsible for conscious, logical thought and inhibition (Odent, 2001). The shift from the new brain to the old brain is facilitated by the release of hormones such as beta-endorphins (Buckley, 2004). Midwives often recognise when a woman's neocortex has shut down because she stops talking and enters a trance-like state (Simkin and Ancheta, 2002). This is often described as the woman 'going into herself'. The shutting down of the neocortex indicates high levels of beta-endorphins and oxytocin and is therefore a good sign that the labour hormones are working well.

The hormonal control of labour and birth is a complex and finely tuned system which has been proven over generations to be 'safe and efficient for the vast majority of women' (Buckley, 2004: 204). When women are frightened, or feel unsafe, however, a surge of adrenaline

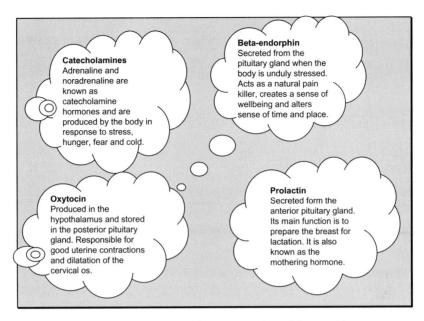

Figure 2.3 Key functions of labour hormones. Adapted from Buckley (2004).

is produced, causing labour to slow down or stop (Gaskin, 2004; Robertson, 2000). Adrenaline production can be triggered by environmental factors and this fact supports the observation that labour dystocia is known to occur more frequently in hospital (Walsh, 1999; Odent, 2001; Walsh and Downe, 2004). This offers a clear explanation of the reason why home birth can readily be viewed as providing labouring women with an optimal birthing environment where physiological birth is more likely to occur.

The art of midwifery

Every day midwives use knowledge and skills that relate to both the art and science of midwifery practice (Thomas, 2000; Thompson, 2004). In a consultant unit setting, science is the dominant discourse and the art of midwifery is often overlooked (Thompson, 2004). The art of midwifery is the ability 'to help women work in harmony with their bodies and open themselves to give birth' (Kitzinger, 2005: 4). Central to this is the development of a trusting relationship with the woman and her family. This enables the midwife to effectively 'tune in' (Robertson, 2000) or 'connect' (Siddiqui, 1999; Mander, 2001) on an emotional level. A woman will only feel truly supported when an element of trust has been established with her midwife (Kirkham, 2000). We have to be aware that inappropriate actions (such as talking whilst a woman is dealing with a contraction) can be counterproductive in supporting labouring women (Hupcey, 1998).

Practising the art of midwifery relies on the use of traditional midwifery skills. Mander (2001) identifies these as the use of a continual presence, protecting labouring women from harm and providing hands-on comfort and encouragement.

Reflection

As a newly qualified midwife, I can remember trying to put labouring women at their ease by engaging them in light hearted conversation. I would rub women's backs, offer advice and generally try to establish a dialogue. It was only as I became more knowledgeable and confident in my own and women's abilities that I realised my actions were intervening in the birthing process rather than supporting it! I only really began to understand how to support physiological birth when I began working as a community midwife.

Odent (2001) stresses that one of the most important things a birth attendant can do is to create a positive and calm atmosphere. This avoids any disturbance of the delicate hormonal interplay of labour and reduces the need for intervention (Walsh and Downe, 2004). A calming environment is also good for midwives, encouraging them to relax and truly be 'with woman'. In this type of environment, midwives should adopt a positive, unobtrusive presence by staying in the background, responding only to overt and covert signals from the woman in labour (Leap, 2000a). Midwifery presence is not about talking to women but about 'being with woman' and this is acknowledged as an essential skill in the facilitation of normal birth (Siddiqui, 1999; Kirkham, 2000; Leap, 2000a; Page, 2000; Mander, 2001). It can, however, be a difficult skill for many midwives to master as hospital birth encourages midwives to be busy because of the number of tasks that have to be completed (Walsh et al., 2004). At home, it is appropriate to adopt the principle 'the less we do the more we give' (Leap, 2000a). Midwifery presence employs the time-honoured skills of watching, waiting and trusting the woman's ability to give birth (Odent, 1996).

Protecting the birth space

Another traditional skill, fundamental to the art of midwifery practice, is protection. Hospital-based midwives have described how they protect women in normal labour from unnecessary intervention by keeping doctors out of the labour room. Crabtree (2004) found that these midwives frequently acted as a 'buffer' between the woman and environmental factors. Protective approaches are at the very heart of traditional midwifery skills and care (Anderson, 2002). In a woman's home, the use of protective midwifery approaches may include closing the birthing room door, drawing the curtains to maintain privacy or turning off mobile phones or televisions to reduce external stimuli (Box 2.3).

Box 2.3 Practice point: creating the optimal birth environment

- Dim the lights or draw the curtains/blinds.
- Use positive birth language and speak softly.
- Avoid giving advice; aim to create a positive midwifery presence.
- Avoid stimulation of the neocortex by reducing noise and other external stimuli, e.g. where possible use a Pinard stethoscope to auscultate the fetal heart, cover up clocks and clinical equipment.
- Keep procedures and observations to a minimum to maintain oxytocin levels and avoid adrenaline production.
- Ensure the room is warm; consider the use of heat pads.
- Make sure the labouring woman has access to food and drink to avoid adrenaline production.
- Avoid the use of drugs as these disturb normal physiology.
- Consider the use of hydrotherapy.

All of these approaches are aimed at maintaining privacy, creating a place of safety and reducing stimulation of the neocortex.

One of the difficulties with protecting the home birthing space is that women sometimes make decisions that the attending midwife may feel are not conducive to physiological labour and birth, for instance inviting friends and neighbours to a birthing party. It might be possible to reach a compromise if the midwife and the woman have built up a trusting relationship but it is also important to acknowledge that some women will benefit from the support provided by a number of significant others.

Physical and psychological support

Gagnon et al. (1997) describe emotional labour support as reassurance, encouragement and distraction from pain. The ability to provide appropriate 'hands-on' and emotional support is a fundamental midwifery skill (Walters and Kirkham, 1997). The use of hands-on comfort and support aims to help women cope with the emotional, as well as the physical, pain of labour (Leap and Anderson, 2004). Berg et al. (1996) recount how labouring women viewed their midwives as their emotional and physical anchor in coping with pain.

In the western world, the majority of women in hospital use pharmacological analgesia to control the pain of labour (Leap and Anderson, 2004). However, the use of drugs in physiological labour should be avoided because they have a detrimental effect on the delicately balanced hormonal interplay (Buckley, 2004). Leap (2000b) describes two differing approaches to helping women cope with the pain of labour: the 'pain relief' medical paradigm and the 'coping with pain' paradigm, which acknowledges and works with physiological birth. At home, most women give birth without any pharmacological analgesia, possibly because they labour and give birth in a supportive environment. As a home birth midwife you need to suggest strategies which do not disturb normal labour physiology but which help women cope with labour pain. Table 2.2 outlines some coping strategies which may be useful when working within the 'coping with pain' paradigm.

In summary, midwifery skills that enhance physiological birth should be adopted for women who choose to labour and birth their babies at home. Case study 2.3 illustrates the use of traditional midwifery skills and the art of midwifery practice.

Table 2.2 Midwifery approaches to support labouring women coping with pain. Adapted from Simkin, P. and Ancheta, A. (2002).

Type of pain	Helpful strategy/strategies
Woman complains of lower back pain	• Massage her lower back to stimulate endorphin release • Relieve pressure by changing her position, e.g. on all fours, standing leaning over a chair, side lying with one or two pillows under her head • Maternal movement during contractions: hip rocking, lunging with foot on a chair or the floor, camel walking (marching but with hips pushed outwards) • Place a heat pad over the affected area • Hydrotherapy: direct a shower of hot water at her lower back or encourage her to float in a warm bath
Woman complains of lower abdominal or frontal pelvic pain	• Encourage maternal movement: walking, dancing, rocking, etc. • Hydrotherapy: bath if possible – use jug to pour water over her abdomen • Encourage her to stand and clasp her hands together under her 'bump' and to gently pull upwards (abdominal lifting). This movement eases pain in the lower abdomen but can also be used to help correct OP position. • Place a warmed heat pad over affected area
General measures women find helpful	• Hold her during the contraction • Dancing/smooching – play relaxing music • Hand and foot massage

Case study 2.3 Jane's birth story

Jane is in labour with her third child. She is labouring in a small sitting room at the back of her house, her daughter is asleep upstairs. Each time Jane has a contraction she leans over the back of the armchair and sways rhythmically, bending and stretching in time to her contractions. Her partner Richard places a heat pad over her lower back and in between contractions holds Jane in his arms. It is 3 o'clock in the morning. The two midwives sit in the corner of the dimly lit room, one quietly making notes and the other hugging a cup of tea. Every so often one of the midwives walks unobtrusively over to Jane and kneels on the floor to listen to the fetal heart. No one speaks. Over the next few hours Jane's contractions become stronger and more frequent, and she begins to call out 'I can't do this anymore!' With the next contraction Jane makes some expulsive noises and calls for the midwives to help her. One midwife moves closer, touching Jane's arm saying 'You're doing so well – I'm here'. The other quietly and carefully prepares the equipment needed for the birth. As the contractions become stronger and more expulsive Jane squats down on the floor and holds her breath instinctively. The midwife quietly places a waterproof sheet on the floor next to Jane.

All is quiet . . . . . .

The attending midwives smile knowingly and encourage Jane to listen to her body. They sit on the floor next to Jane, with their gloved hands clasped in quiet expectation. With the next contraction Jane tells the midwives that her baby is coming. Jane pushes and the midwife catches the baby's advancing head. With one final push a baby boy is born onto the floor. Jane and Richard gaze down at their newborn son, who begins to cry.

The sun streams through the curtains – the midwives smile and say what a wonderful start to the day!

Reflection exercise

- Write down your feelings about the midwives who were with Jane for her birth.
- Think about the last normal birth you attended and reflect on if/how you used traditional midwifery skills.
- If you did not use traditional midwifery skills, identify why this might be. What stopped you?
- Identify how you can incorporate the 'art' of midwifery into the care of low-risk women.

Summary

This chapter has identified the fact that more than 20% of pregnant women would seriously consider having their babies at home. It is also possible to conclude that a geographical variation in home birth rates exists because of the way that maternity services are organised and the negative attitudes of a number of healthcare professionals. Stephens (2005) suggests that an increase in the rate of home birth might help in the recruitment and retention of midwives and also establish midwives as the true experts in normal birth.

Midwives need to be proactive in raising home birth rates by offering home birth to all women with low-risk pregnancies. This should be coupled with awareness that some women may not be able to make an informed decision until the birth is imminent. The place of birth should therefore be discussed throughout pregnancy in order to facilitate real choice.

The need to increase alternatives to consultant-based units has been recognised in the National Service Framework (DH, 2004) for maternity care and a woman's right to choose home birth is supported by the RCM (2002) and NMC (2006b). Current research evidence identifies that home birth is a safe option for women with low-risk pregnancies and should be offered to all suitable women.

The introduction of the National Service Framework for maternity care may herald the start of political pressure to develop a system of care that supports low-risk birth and midwifery practice. However, if maternity services and midwives fail to develop and promote home birth services then true choice for pregnant women and the art of midwifery may be lost.

Key points

- Key research evidence exists to support the safety of home birth.
- The wide geographical variations in home birth rates may be linked to the attitudes of doctors and midwives and the regional organisation of maternity services.
- An evidence-based framework can be applied by community midwives to promote choice in the place of birth.
- Midwives have contractual and professional obligations when an NHS trust withdraws its home birth service.
- Physiological birth is facilitated through the art of midwifery.

References

AIMS (2006) Association for improvements in maternity services. http://www.aims.org.uk (accessed September 2006).

Albany Midwifery Practice (2003) Birth statistics. http://www.albanymidwives. org.uk (accessed July 2006).

Allison, J. (1996) *Delivered at Home*. Nelson Thornes, Oxford.

Anderson, T. (2002) Out of the laboratory: back to the darkened room. *MIDIRS Midwifery Digest*, **12** (1), 65–69.

Andrews, A. (2004) Home birth experience 2: births/postnatal reflections. *British Journal of Midwifery*, **14** (12), 552–557.

BBC News (2004) Midwife sacked after home birth. 22 August 2004 http:// newsbbc.co.uk/health. 22nd August 2004. http://news.bbc.co.uk/1/health/ (accessed September 2006).

Berg, M., Lundgren, I., Hermansson, E. and Wahlberg, V. (1996) Women's encounter with the midwife during childbirth. *Midwifery*, **12**, 11–15.

BirthChoiceUK (2006) Where to have your baby? http://www.birthchoiceuk. com (accessed January 2006).

Buckley, S. (2004) Undisturbed birth — nature's hormonal blue print for safety, ease and ecstacy. *MIDIRS Midwifery Digest*, **14** (2), 203–209.

Cluett, E.R. and Bluff, R. (2000) *Principles and Practice of Research in Midwifery*. Blackwell Science, Oxford.

Crabtree, S. (2004) Midwives constructing normal birth. In: *Normal Childbirth: Evidence and Debate* (ed. S. Downe), Chapter 6. Churchill Livingstone, London.

Davis, L. (2004) 'Allowed' shouldn't be allowed! *MIDIRS Midwifery Digest*, **14** (2), 151–156.

Davis-Floyd, R.E. (1992) *Birth as an American Rite of Passage*. University of California, Berkley, California.

Davis-Floyd, R.E. and Sargent, C. (eds) (1997) *Childbirth and Authoritative Knowledge*. California Press, California.

DeVries, R. and Barroso, R. (1997) Midwives among the machines: recreating midwifery in the late twentieth century. In: *Midwives Society and Childbirth: Debates and Controversies in the Modern Period* (eds H. Marland and A.M. Rafferty), Chapter 12. Routledge, London.

DH (1993) *Changing Childbirth*. HMSO, London.

DH (2004) *National Service Framework for Children, Young People and Maternity Services*. Department of Health, London.

DH (2005) NHS maternity statistics, England: 2003–2004. www.dh.gov.uk/ publications and statistics (accessed September 2006).

DH/PCFM (2007) *Maternity Matters: Choice, Access and Continuity of Care in a Safe Service*. Department of Health/Partnership for Children, Families and Maternity, London.

Edwards, N. (2005) *Birthing Autonomy: Women's Experiences of Home Births*. Routledge, London.

Enkin, M., Keirse, M., Neilson, J., Crowther, C., et al. (2000) *Guide to Effective Care in Pregnancy and Childbirth*, 3rd edn. Oxford University Press, Oxford.

Fisher, J.R.W. (2002) Difficult deliveries, disenfranchised grief and delayed trauma reactions. In: *The Fertile Imagination: Narratives of Reproduction* (eds

M. Kirkham, J.M. Maher and K. Tourney-Souter). The La Trobe University English Review **18** (2), 39–58.

Floyd, L. (1995) Community midwives views and experiences of homebirth. *Midwifery* **11** (1), 3–10.

Gagnon, I.M., Waghorn, K. and Covell, C. (1997) A randomised trial of one-to-one support of women in labour. *Birth*, **24** (2), 71–77.

Gaskin, I. (2004) Smile for your sphincter. *The Practising Midwife*, **7** (10), 4–5.

Gibbons, J. and Thomson, A.M. (2001) Women's expectations and experiences of childbirth. *Midwifery*, **17** (4), 302–313.

Green, J.M., Coupland, V.A. and Kitzinger, J.V. (1998) *Great Expectations: A Prospective Study of Women's Expectation and Experiences of Childbirth*. Books for Midwives, Hale.

Hodnett, E.D., Lowe, N., Hannah, M.E., et al. (2002) Effectiveness of nurses as providers of birth labour support in North American Hospitals: a RCT. *Journal of the American Medical Association*, **288**, 1373–1381.

Hosein, M.C. (1998) Homebirth: is it a real option? *British Journal of Midwifery*, **6** (6), 370–373.

Hupcey, J.E. (1998) Clarifying the social support theory. *Journal of Advanced Nursing*, **27** (6), 1231–1241.

Johnson, R. (2000) Beyond defensive practice: promoting quality, promoting normality, in, RCM. *The Rising Caesarean Section Rate: Causes and Effects for Public Health*. Conference report, November, joint publication RCM, RCOG, NCT, London.

Kinsey, J. (2005) Home birth: safe as houses? *The Practising Midwife*, **8** (7), 27–29.

Kirkham, M. (2000) How we relate? In: *The Midwife Mother Relationship* (ed. M. Kirkham), Chapter 11. Macmillan Press, London.

Kirkham, M. (2003) A cycle of empowerment: the enabling culture of birth centres. *The Practising Midwife*, **6** (11), 12–15.

Kitzinger, S. (2000) Sheila Kitzinger's letter from Europe: home birth matters. *Birth*, **27** (1), 61–62.

Kitzinger, S. (2005) Midwifery degraded. *The Practising Midwife*, **8** (8), 4–5.

Leap, N. (2000a) The less we do, the more we give. In: *The Midwife Mother Relationship* (ed. M. Kirkham), Chapter 2. Macmillan Press, London.

Leap, N. (2000b) Towards a midwifery perspective. *MIDIRS Midwifery Digest*, **10** (1), 49–53.

Leap, N. and Anderson, T. (2004) The role of pain in normal birth and the empowerment of women. In: *Normal Childbirth: Evidence and Debate* (ed. S. Downe), Chapter 1. Churchill Livingstone, London.

Lord Hunt of Kings Heath (2000) *Hansard*, 20 December: column 734.

Mander, R. (2001) *Supportive Care and Midwifery*. Blackwell Science, Oxford.

McNabb, M. (1997) Hormonal interactions in labour. In: *Mayes Midwifery: A Textbook for Midwives* (ed. B. Sweet), 12th edn., pp. 234–261. Baillere Tindall, London.

Morison, S., Hauck, Y., Percival, P. and McMurray, A. (1998) Constructing a home birth environment through assuming control. *Midwifery*, **14** (4), 233–241.

NCT (2001) *Home birth in the United Kingdom*. National Childbirth Trust, London.

NICE (2006) *Draft Intrapartum Guideline*. National Institute for Clinical Excellence, London. http://www.nice.org.uk (accessed September 2006).

NMC (2004a) *Code of Professional Conduct*. Nursing and Midwifery Council, London.

NMC (2004b) *Midwives Rules and Standards*. Nursing and Midwifery Council, London.

NMC (2006b) *Midwives and Home Birth*, NMC circular 8. Nursing and Midwifery Council, London.

Odent, M. (1996) Why labouring women don't need support. *Mothering*, **80** (Autumn), 47–51.

Odent, M. (2001) New reasons and new ways to study birth physiology. *The International Journal of Gynecology and Obstetrics*, **75**, S39–S45.

Office of National Statistics (2004) Birth trends: birth by birth order in England and Wales (September 2002). http://www.statistics.gov.uk/birth (accessed September 2005).

Olsen, O. and Jewell, M.D. (2002) Home versus hospital birth (Cochrane review). *The Cochrane Library*, Issue 1. Update Software, Oxford.

Page, L. (2000) Putting science and sensitivity in practice. In: *The New Midwifery: Science and Sensitivity in Practice* (ed. L. Page), Chapter 1. Churchill Livingstone, London.

Perkins, B. (2004) *The Medical Delivery Business: Health Reform, Childbirth, and the Economic Order*. Rutgers University Press, London.

Queniart, A. (1992) Risky business: medical definitions of pregnancy. In: *Anatomy of Gender: Women's Struggle for the Body* (eds D.H. Currie and V. Raoul). Carleton University Press, Ontario, Canada.

RCM (2002) *Position Paper 25: Home Birth*. Royal College of Midwives, London.

Rayhald, I. (1545) *The Byrth of Mankyinde*. London.

Robertson, A. (2000) *The Midwife Companion: The Art of Support During Birth*. ACE graphics, Camperdown, Austrailia.

Rowe-Murray, H.J. and Fisher, J.R.W. (2002) Baby friendly hospital practices: caesarean section is a persistent barrier to early initiation of breast feeding. *Birth*, **29**, 124–131.

Sackett, D.L., Strauss, S.E., Richardson, W.S., Rosenburg, W. and Haynes, R.B. (2002) *Evidence Based Medicine. How to Practise and Teach EBM*. Churchill Livingstone, Edinburgh.

Siddiqui, J. (1999) The therapeutic relationship in midwifery. *British Journal of Midwifery*, **7** (2), 111–114.

Simkin, P. (1992) Just another day in a woman's life? Part two: nature and consistence of women's long-term memories of their birth experiences. *Birth*, **19** (1), 64–81.

Simkin, P. and Ancheta, A. (2002) *The Labour Progress Handbook*. Blackwell Science, Oxford.

Singh, D. and Newburn, M. (2000) *Access to Maternity Information and Support: The Needs and Experiences of Pregnant Women and New Mothers*. National Childbirth Trust, London.

Stephens, L. (2005) Worrying truth behind home birth figures. *British Journal of Midwifery*, **13** (1), 4–5.

Tew, M. (1998) *Safer Childbirth? A Critical History of Maternity Care*. 3rd revised edition. Free Association Books, London.

Thomas, G. (2000) Be nice and don't drop the baby. In: *The New Midwifery: Science and Sensitivity in Practice* (ed. L. Page), Chapter 9. Churchill Livingstone, London.

Thompson, F.E. (2004) *Mothers and Midwives: The Ethical Journey*. Books for Midwives, London.

Wagner, M. (1995) *Pursuing the Birth Machine: The Search for Appropriate Birth Technology*. ACE Graphics, Sydney.

Walsh, D. (1999) An ethnographic study of women's experience of partnership caseload midwifery: the professional as a friend. *Midwifery*, **15**, 165–176.

Walsh, D. (2000) Evidence-based care, series 1: birth environment. *British Journal of Midwifery*, **8** (6), 351–355.

Walsh, D. (2002) The impact of the birth environment. *Research Update: Report from Preston National Symposium on the Current Evidence Base for Normal Birth*. http://www.midwivesonline.com/preston.htm (accessed October 2005).

Walsh, D. and Downe, S. (2004) A systematic review of free-standing midwifery led units and birth centres. *Birth*, **31** (3), 222–229.

Walsh, D., El-Nemer, A. and Downe, S. (2004) Risk, safety and the study of physiological birth. In: *Normal Childbirth: Evidence and Debate* (ed. S. Downe), Chapter 7. Churchill Livingstone, London.

Walters, D. and Kirkham M. (1997) Support and control in labour: doulas and midwives. In: *Reflections on Midwifery* (eds M. Kirkham and E.R. Perkins), Chapter 5. Baillière Tindall, London.

Woodcock, H.C., Read, A.W., Bower, C., Stanby, F.J. and Moore, D. (1994) A matched cohort study of planned home and hospital births in Western Australia 1981–1987. *Midwifery*, **10**, 125–135.

Home birth against advice

Elaine Newell

The number of women who choose to give birth at home against the advice of a healthcare professional is relatively few. The impact that such a choice will have on a woman, and the professional and personal conflicts which are often experienced by the midwives caring for her in such circumstances, cannot be underestimated.

Carter (2004) cites a number of issues which, to the professional, may present a controversial choice for a woman in relation to home birth. These can be predominantly considered in two main categories. Firstly, some women make choices which are deemed contrary to the advice of the individual professional or professional group. This may be because the woman's choice contravenes local or national policy or guidance, or because it conflicts with the opinion or evidential knowledge held by the professional. The professional then holds the belief that the woman and her baby are at greater actual or perceived risk. Such examples might include a request for home birth following previous caesarean section or a breech birth at home. Secondly, the woman's request for a home birth is not covered by local service arrangements, i.e. the local trust does not provide a home birth service.

This chapter seeks to undertake a pragmatic review of the legislative framework which exists around home birth and will analyse some of the issues which underpin this, such as the debate around informed choice. It will also consider the practical support available for community midwives when supporting women who choose to have a controversial home birth.

The concept of risk

The assessment of risk is generally a systematic process undertaken within a framework of individual trust policies. These are supported by national guidance provided by the National Institute for Clinical Excellence (NICE), the Clinical Negligence Scheme for Trusts (CNST) and current best evidence. In considering choices which are contrary to policy, guidance, evidence or personally held values and beliefs, it is important to consider the models of care which impact upon our assessment and acceptance of risk.

Walsh (2006) discusses the issue of risk and maternal health to explore the contrasting views and potential conflict which can arise when applying two differing models of care within a maternity setting. He points to the 'technocratic model' which exerts the view that childbirth is only normal in retrospect. The primary focus within this model is on outcomes. It monitors outcomes by 'what goes wrong' through emphasis on mortality and morbidity statistics. It is dependent on medical interventions to prevent deviations from the norm, regardless of the likelihood of risk. Walsh (2006) suggests that this model, commonly used throughout maternity care, actually predisposes women to iatrogenic risk. Clinical iatrogenesis is a term used to describe the risks associated with the direct consequences of medical treatment or intervention (Illich, 2001). Walsh (2006) goes on to explore an alternative approach to risk management in discussing the 'social' model of care. This model focuses less on the avoidance of risk, and more on the 'promotion of efficacy'. This places greater weight on the risks and issues important to women as opposed to risks based on professional beliefs. Consider the example in Box 3.1.

Box 3.1 Perceptions of risk

The midwife, who is measuring risk in terms of the probability of adverse outcome, may feel that it is highly unsuitable for a woman with a previous caesarean section (CS) to give birth at home, based on her/his knowledge that a percentage of women with a previous CS will sustain a uterine rupture. The woman, however, may have previously required an operative delivery due to 'failure to progress'. She may have laboured on a busy delivery suite where one-to-one midwifery care was unavailable. Her valid perceptions are those of limited support in labour and poor continuity of care. As a result she requested epidural anaesthesia, was rendered immobile and required augmentation of her labour.

The woman might understandably feel that the risks of another labour experience in hospital, with limited support and very little control of her birth process, is too much of a risk to take again. In her view, the very real probability of encountering a similar experience if she agrees to a hospital birth far outweighs the potential risks presented by the midwife.

Nolan (2002) advocates the application and use of similar themes, such as continuity of care and carer, in encouraging service providers to view the application of social models as preventative, rather than obstructive, approaches to care. This view is supported by Campbell and MacFarlane (1994), who argue that the iatrogenic effects associated with institutional birth (i.e. the risks of being unable to access one-to-one care in labour and greater exposure to the risks associated with increased medical intervention) are often overlooked when discussing birth at home. In real terms, what the woman considers as an important risk avoidance strategy (care in a familiar environment, the certainty of one-to-one care, the presence of her family) may be diametrically opposed to the risk avoidance approaches applied by the professional. It is this issue which often underpins conflicts when dealing with women who request home birth against professional advice. Fielder et al. (2004) discuss the ways in which professionals have a tendency to work in opposites. For example,

- home/hospital
- safe/unsafe
- normal/abnormal.

Fielder and colleagues suggest that these opposites tend to be constructed as positive versus negative or good versus bad. They imply a value judgement which separates the unacceptable to place it outside the social norm for a particular group.

Safety is often viewed by professionals as an absolute concept when, in fact, this is rarely the case. The DH (1993) states that 'safety is not an absolute concept . . . It is part of a greater picture of health and well being'. It is often extremely difficult for midwives to separate their deeply rooted beliefs and values regarding safety (which, it could be argued, arise from a technocratic model of care) from those of the broader, more socially rooted values which may be held by women. As a result, it is imperative that professionals seek to determine the values and priorities of each individual woman when assessing risk and discussing place of birth. Discussion regarding potential risks and priorities should take place early in pregnancy so that plans to support both the woman and the midwife can be well thought through and clearly communicated.

NHS trust obligation and the provision of home birth services

Maternity services in all four countries of the UK were subject to extensive review in the 1990s (DH, 1993). Documents were subsequently produced by all four government health departments containing key recommendations, all of which placed women at the centre of maternity care and emphasised the importance of choice for women. This included choice regarding place of birth. However, there is no specific legal provision for home birth under the requirement of the National Health Service Act (Great Britain, 1977). Section 1 of the Act imposes a general duty upon the Secretary of State to provide a national health service. The way in which the service is delivered is subject to his or her statutory discretion:

> 'It is the Secretary of State's duty to provide throughout England and Wales, to such extent as he feels necessary, to meet all reasonable requirements:
> (a) hospital accommodation; (b) other accommodation for the purpose of any service provided under this Act; (c) medical, dental, nursing and ambulance services; (d) other such facilities for the care of expectant and nursing mothers as he considers are appropriate as part of the Health Service.' National Health Service Act (Great Britain, 1977), Section 3(1)

Whilst there is no statutory duty placed on trusts to provide any specific aspect of maternity services, trusts are expected to provide services which respond to local need. Government policies in all the four countries of the UK promote choice for women in relation to place of birth and embrace the philosophy of woman-centred care. This has been a consistent message. At the Royal College of Midwives Conference in 2001, Alan Milburn the Secretary of State for Health made the following statement:

> 'In some areas, home births are widely available to women: in others they are not. Our standard must be to end the lottery in childbirth choices so that women in all parts of the country, not just some, have greater choice, including the choice of a home birth'. Cited in the report of House of Commons Health Committee (2003)

The *National Service Framework for Children, Young People and Maternity Services* (DH, 2004) recommends that maternity care providers and PCTs ensure that the range of antenatal, intrapartum and postnatal services available locally constitute real choice for women (including home birth). In short, trusts are not statutorily obliged to provide home birth services, but arguably it would be against government policy for them not to do so.

Whilst, as previously mentioned, the right of trusts to provide a home birth service is not one based in statute, women in the UK have an absolute right to give birth at home simply because there is no legal compulsion for a woman to attend hospital for birth if she is mentally competent. The exception to this would be women prisoners, some minors and adults who lack mental capacity. The topic of capacity will be explored later in this chapter.

Are midwives obliged to attend a home birth?

Both the professional and contractual obligations of the midwife must be explored when considering her or his position in relation to attendance at a home birth. Professional obligations are outlined in the NMC rules and codes (NMC, 2004a, b). In meeting the statutory professional regulations and in keeping with the requirements for self regulation, a midwife is required to meet the ethical standards set out in the *Code of Professional Conduct* and the *Midwives' Rules*. It is explicit within these standards that midwives should:

- offer women accessible, evidence-based information
- respect a woman's choice
- support women in their choice (NMC, 2006).

The *Midwives' Rules* (NMC, 2004b) apply to all midwives undertaking their professional duties. For the majority of midwives these professional duties will be carried under a contractual obligation with an NHS trust. Rule 6:1 clearly states that all practising midwives have a responsibility to provide midwifery care for women and their babies during pregnancy, labour and the postnatal period. The associated NMC guidance specifies that when a woman rejects advice, the midwife should continue to provide the best possible care, seeking support from other members of the healthcare team as necessary (NMC, 2004b). The *Code of Professional Conduct* (NMC, 2004a) continues this theme to assert that 'you must respect patients' and clients' autonomy – their right to decide whether to undergo any healthcare intervention – even when a refusal may result in harm or death to themselves or a fetus unless a court of law orders to the contrary'.

There have been reports in the midwifery press (Flint, 2004) of occasions where the intention of the woman to give birth at home conflicts with the demands of the employer, i.e. the trust has stipulated that it cannot provide a home birth service but the woman refuses to go into hospital for her birth. Whilst this is an extremely rare occurrence, it does place the midwife in a very difficult position.

The NMC (2006) circular *Midwives and Home Birth* declares that, should conflict arise between a service provider and a woman regarding place of birth, the midwife still has a duty to provide care. Many midwives believe that it is their statutory duty to attend a woman in labour. Rosser (1998) discusses this in greater detail and states that, in actual fact, the duty upon a midwife to attend a woman in labour is part of her contractual duty with the trust for whom she works – and not part of a statutory obligation. Rosser states that if a community midwife is called to attend a woman in labour, she does so because, in the course of her employment, she has accepted the responsibility to do so and has a contractual duty to attend.

In the rare event of an NHS trust withdrawing the provision of home birth services, the midwife would no longer have a contractual duty to attend a woman at home. Indeed, by doing so, she/he would be acting outside of her/his employment contract and would not be indemnified to provide care because she/he would be working independently of the trust. The exception to this would of course be those independent midwives who are working outside of NHS contracts. Independent midwives will be bound by professional rules and codes and contractual agreements with individual women.

When conflict arises, it is essential that the midwife discusses the emerging issues with a manager in the first instance and then the involvement of a supervisor of midwives should be sought. If the conflict cannot be resolved, the midwife should inform the local supervising authority midwifery officer (LSAMO). Magill-Cuerden (2005) suggests that the maternity service provider is likely to uphold guidance given by the local supervising authority. The midwife may also wish to seek advice from her trade union or professional representative.

The Royal College of Midwives (RCM, 2002) recognise that there may be emergency situations, for instance during extreme staffing shortages or unplanned peaks in activity, where it is necessary to focus all resources on the hospital service, temporarily suspending the home birth service. They advise that this would be viewed as a significant breach of good practice and trusts would be expected to review and resolve such decisions as a matter of urgency. In such a scenario, women may still decide to give birth at home. Where it is envisaged that this will occur, it is imperative that maternity service managers work closely with midwives and supervisors to develop robust contingency plans. These plans should support community midwives and offer clear advice regarding their position should such a situation occur.

Woman-centred care and controversial home birth

The philosophy of woman-centred care is one which, as previously mentioned, underpins government policy relating to the provision of maternity care. Fundamental to this philosophy is the need to ensure that women have the opportunity to make an equal contribution to the planning and delivery of their own care and that maternity services are designed and shaped to meet their needs. Giving women information in order to inform their choices and enabling them to control and contribute to decisions regarding their care are key principles of autonomy and central to a woman-centred approach (DH, 1993; RCM, 2001). Autonomy has been defined as:

> 'The capacity to think, decide and then act upon a decision freely and independently' Gillon (1986)

Gill and Stirratt (2003) suggest that true autonomy cannot be exercised without reference to other moral agents, such as relationships and community. This effectively means that when she exercises her choice relating to home birth a woman will weigh the information she possesses against her own set of values and beliefs, measuring what is important to her personally. She can then use this information, alongside that gleaned from the professional, to determine and shape her decision.

Informed choice

Informed choice is crucial to a woman's ability to make decisions about her care. It is the word 'informed' – often liberally used by professionals – which is the common denominator between choice, decisions, consent or refusal. The NMC (2004a) directs professionals to ensure that 'information should be accurate, truthful and presented in such a way as to make it easily understood'.

Every midwife has both a legal and professional obligation to provide care for her clients. This is referred to in law as a 'duty of care'. The law defines duty of care in the health context as that being owed to all of the clients that a midwife has a contractual responsibility for, within the terms of her employment (Dimond, 2006). The duty of care includes a duty to communicate with a client and inform her about benefits and risks. Failure to communicate information relating to treatment and care may be considered negligent, or as a failure in that duty of care if the client subsequently suffers harm as a result of missing or misleading information.

Ley (1988, in Wilson and Symon, 2002) identifies three particular problems which commonly affect communication and inhibit informed choice:

- The presentation of information in a manner that is too difficult for women to understand.
- Failure to recognise that a number of women may lack even a basic knowledge of the anatomy and physiology of the reproductive process.
- Failure to identify and eliminate many of the old wives tales and hearsay which underpin and shape women's views and expectations.

Kirkham et al. (2002) argue that informed choice within current healthcare provision is simply rhetoric. They assert that a choice can only be made when an individual has had sufficient access to information and knowledge to underpin a reasoned decision. Kirkham continues to argue that the information made available by midwives and obstetricians is often framed in a way which supports professionally defined 'right choices' and Levy (2004) identifies ways in which midwives act as gatekeepers of information. Kirkham and Stapleton (2004) demonstrate how issues such as the power and influence of the medical model of care, pressures of time and the need to conform to hierarchical norms will all affect how professionals exchange information. All midwives need to be mindful of the influences imposed by the culture in which they practise. They must recognise that enabling choice is a very complex process if they are truly aiming to facilitate an informed and balanced discussion regarding place of birth (Box 3.2).

Box 3.2 Practice point

Nolan (2002) suggests that there are a number of key questions which should underpin the information given to women. These simple questions can easily be translated into discussion with the woman who is considering a home birth against advice.

- What are the benefits?
- What might be the drawbacks?
- What are the alternatives?
- What will happen if we do nothing?
- How long do we have to make a decision?

A reasonable standard of information

Professionals often struggle with what constitutes a reasonable standard of information. The courts determine the level of information that needs to be discussed with a patient by using the Bolam test (Box 3.3). A practitioner would not be deemed negligent if his/her treatment or standard of care conformed to that of a reasonable body of opinion held by practitioners skilled in the field in question.

Box 3.3 The Bolam test

John Bolam was a psychiatric patient undergoing electroconvulsive therapy (ECT). He was not warned of the risk of fractures due to convulsions during treatment. Mr Bolam was given no muscle relaxants, neither was he restrained during treatment. He subsequently sustained bilateral fractures of the acetabulum as a direct result of the ECT.

In considering the case, the judge determined that the test of negligence be:

'the standard of the ordinary skilled man exercising and professing to have that special skill.'

During the case, a number of other doctors testified that they would have treated Bolam in the same way. The judge determined therefore that a reasonable body of doctors would not have acted any differently and Bolam's doctor was found not guilty of negligence.

Bolam vs Friern Hospital Management Committee (1957) 1WLR 582

The Bolam ruling was subsequently endorsed in the Sidaway case (Sidaway vs. Bethlem Royal Hospital Governors 1985). However, this also stated that it was open to the courts to determine whether information regarding a particular risk was so obviously necessary that it would be negligent not to provide it, even if a responsible body of experts would not have done so. Whilst standards set by professionals will have a significant influence, it will ultimately rest with the courts to determine what must be considered reasonable in terms of giving information (DH, 2001).

Social inequalities often mean that clients who are less well educated, less articulate or challenged by language difficulties may struggle with information given to them by a healthcare professional. Communication barriers caused by inequalities are frequently cited by the *Confidential Enquiry* reports (Lewis, 2004) as major risks in the provision of health care. Midwives are directed by the NMC (2004b) to work in partnership with a woman and her family, discussing matters with her in full, to enable her to make decisions about her care based on individual needs and preferences. Professional knowledge inevitably creates a position of power and the potential for inequalities in the provision of knowledge is very real. Davis (1994) suggests that the provision of information requires a change in the relationship between clients and professionals in order to redress the balance of power, from one of control over professional knowledge to one where knowledge and decision making are equally shared. Informed consent acknowledges that the client has the right to autonomy and self-determination. It also presumes that clients have the capacity or competence to make decisions regarding their care.

What is capacity?

Providing they have the mental capacity, the law recognises that every individual has the absolute right to make decisions relating to their plans for care. Capacity, or competence to make decisions, has been defined as:

> ... 'the ability to comprehend and retain information material to a decision, especially as to the consequences of having or not having the intervention in question, and must be able to use and weigh this information in the decision making process'. DH (2001)

In the majority of cases, women will have the capacity to make decisions regarding their place of birth, even when those decisions are in direct contrast with the knowledge, principles, values or beliefs of the healthcare profession. The DH acknowledges that the capacity of an individual must be considered distinctly from any judgement that a healthcare professional might profess in relation to the basis of a client's decision:

'The patient is entitled to make a decision which is based on their own religious beliefs or value system, even if it is perceived by others to be irrational, as long as the patient understands what is entailed in their decision. Capacity should not be confused with a healthcare professional's assessment of the reasonableness of the patient's decision.' DH (2001)

In practice, the only women who would lack capacity are those who are deemed unable to do so under the Mental Capacity Act (Great Britain, 2005). This Act was partially enforced in April 2007 and follows a number of cases related to court-authorised caesarean sections. The Act states that a person must be assumed to have capacity unless it has been otherwise established. A woman should not be treated as unable to make a decision (or lacking in capacity) just because her decision is considered to be unwise. The Act recognises that a person is only lacking in capacity if at the time in question she or he is unable to make a decision for herself because of an 'impairment of or a disturbance in the functioning of the mind or brain'. If the refusal of a mentally competent adult were overruled, this would constitute trespass to the person (Dimond, 2006).

The role of the supervisor of midwives

Professional guidance places emphasis on seeking advice and support from supervisors of midwives (SoM) in cases where women express a desire to give birth at home against advice (RCM, 2002; NMC, 2006). So what can the SoM actually do? Guidance contained within the NMC rules state that the role of the SoM is to:

'Protect the public by empowering midwives and midwifery students to practise safely and effectively . . . when midwives are faced with a situation where they feel they need support and advice, the Supervisor of Midwives acts as a resource. Supervisors can assist in discussions with women where concerns are expressed regarding the provision of care'. NMC (2004b)

It is important to be clear that it is not the role of the SoM to dissuade the woman from her reasoned choice. The NMC Standards (NMC, 2006) cite one of the roles of the SoM as being that of an 'advocate for the right of all women to make informed choices and contribute to decision making relating to their care'. The SoM should focus on ensuring that the woman has received sufficient information regarding the choices available – either directly or by acting as a resource to the midwife caring for her.

Many NHS trusts have adopted a policy where an SoM will visit all women who express a desire to have a home birth against advice but blanket policies can be unhelpful and each situation should be assessed on its own merit. The SoM and the midwife should give careful consideration to their approach because the woman may view a visit by the SoM as a further attempt by professionals to coerce her into a plan of care that she is opposed to. If an SoM plans to visit a woman, she or he must make certain that the woman has a clear understanding of the role.

More often than not, it is the midwife who is in need of an SoM's support when caring for a woman who chooses controversial home birth. In circumstances where the professionals believe the woman to be placing herself at great risk, midwives can often experience a great deal of personal anxiety and stress. The impact that this has on community midwives cannot be underestimated (Box 3.4).

Box 3.4 The role of the supervisor of midwives

- Direct the midwife to appropriate sources of support.
- Facilitate reflection.
- Promote discussion and debate.
- Debrief the midwife following completion of the case.
- Direct the midwife towards professional legislation in cases where the midwife expresses the desire to 'opt out' of providing care.
- Encourage the midwife to share valuable experiences with colleagues, to provide mutual support and shared learning.
- Advise and direct the midwife in relation to practical and practice issues, such as appropriate documentation, developing plans for care, accessing legal advice and ensuring that the midwife is appropriately skilled to deal with any emergency situations arising.

At the time of writing, the draft NICE (2006) guidelines for intrapartum care advocate that an SoM must be involved if a woman is deemed to have risk factors and wishes to give birth in any location outside of a consultant unit. As previously stated, the extent of the SoM's involvement should be determined on an individual basis. In some cases, it may be necessary for the SoM to attend a home birth; however, access to the patient's home remains at the behest of the woman and it is essential that the reasons for the SoM's attendance are made clear. In all cases, the SoM must remain accessible. This usually requires a commitment to a 24-hour on-call service for the duration of the woman's likely delivery period.

The SoM should also act as a conduit for information. In instances where conflicts arise between the manager and the midwife (i.e. where the trust has withdrawn support for home birth) the SoM can negotiate with the manager to act as an advocate for both midwife and client.

Documentation

Full, detailed and contemporaneous documentation is a vital aspect of care in any case. For the majority of midwives, its importance assumes even greater validity when clients make controversial choices regarding their care. Inconsistent or poor record keeping is frequently cited as a key factor contributing to litigation or poor outcomes. The standard of record keeping is recognised as being directly related to the standard of care provided (NMC, 2005) (Box 3.5).

Box 3.5 Practice point: documentation

When caring for women who choose a controversial home birth, it might be useful for community midwives to discuss and document the following:

- Why does the woman want a home birth – what are her priorities and personal motives?
- What would represent a positive or negative outcome for her personally?
- What are the professionally assessed risks and associated potential outcomes for the woman and her baby?
- What are the limitations regarding the ability to predict outcome?
- How easy/difficult is it to predict potential outcomes?
- What factors might prevent the woman achieving her desired outcomes?
- What level of care can the woman reasonably expect to receive during the labour and birth at home?
- What are the limitations of this care? What are the advantages?
- If the woman proceeds with her wish for home birth, what circumstances might necessitate transfer to hospital?
- What strategies might be put in place if things do not proceed according to the agreed birth plan?
- What are the alternatives – hospital birth, birth centre, DOMINO scheme? What are the advantages, disadvantages and limitations of these – particular to the individual woman?
- What information has been given to the woman to support her decision-making (leaflets, websites, sign-posting to other resources such as the NCT, etc.)?
- The woman must be advised that she can change her mind at any time.

Comprehensive record keeping forms part of the midwife's duty of care. The statutory duty in relation to record keeping is clearly stated within the *Midwives' Rules* and the supporting guidance states:

'Your records relating to the care of women and babies are an essential aspect of practice to aid communication between you, the woman and others who are providing care. They demonstrate whether you have provided an appropriate standard of care to a woman or baby.' NMC (2005)

The NMC (2005) *Guidelines for Records and Record Keeping* make the important point that records should be written with the involvement of the woman, thus demonstrating clear evidence that the care has been jointly planned. When caring for women who choose home birth against advice, this is extremely useful. If facilitated appropriately, this evident involvement should allow women to feel that they have contributed and to feel that they are in control of their own birth plans. Equally, it will enable midwives to clearly capture the information that they have given and the subsequent views of the women they are caring for.

Can the midwife be held responsible if problems arise during a home birth?

In supporting women who intend to give birth at home against advice, community midwives are often extremely anxious that they are at greater risk of liability should a complication and adverse outcome occur. In order for a midwife to be deemed negligent, the burden of proof is with the plaintiff (the person making the allegation). 'Negligence' is the term used to describe an action or failure to act (omission) that breaches a duty of care and subsequently results in harm (Dimond, 2006). In order to prove that the midwife breached her duty of care the plaintiff must prove:

- that harm occurred
- that the midwife had a duty of care
- that the duty of care was breached
- that the breach of duty was the direct cause of the harm suffered.

It is clear that the midwife has a duty of care to her client, regardless of whether or not she agrees with the decisions or choices the woman has made. This duty arises in most cases from her contractual obligation to provide care. Jones and Jenkins (2003) state that midwives can only be held responsible for their own actions or omissions: they cannot be held accountable for complications beyond their control.

Consider the fictional Case studies 3.1 and 3.2.

Case study 3.1 Anna's home birth

Anna is expecting her second baby. Her first was born by caesarean section for 'failure to progress'. She has chosen to give birth at home this time because she feels that the benefit of one-to-one care by a midwife will increase her chance of a vaginal birth. Her midwife, Kelly, discussed the options for care early in pregnancy and provided Anna with information relating to the potential risks and benefit of home and hospital birth. Kelly has discussed the normal practice for monitoring the fetal heart in labour with Anna and has provided her with the reasons and evidence to support this. Kelly has also discussed the complications which might necessitate transfer into hospital. Kelly has documented her discussions fully, following advice from her SoM. She has maintained her mandatory training requirements relating to fetal heart monitoring and has attended training to update her skills in the management of emergency situations.

During Anna's labour Kelly records her observations of the fetal heart every 15 minutes. She notices a reduction in the baseline fetal heart rate and some late decelerations. Having discussed her concerns with Anna, she immediately contacts the consultant unit and makes arrangements for transfer. The time from phoning 999 to arrival at the consultant unit is 30 minutes. On arrival at the delivery suite Anna needs an emergency caesarean section and her baby is delivered requiring extensive resuscitation. His prognosis is poor.

Kelly's documentation demonstrates that she has taken all possible steps to inform Anna of potential risks. She has also monitored the fetal heart appropriately during labour and made a good decision to transfer Anna urgently, as soon as she suspected a deviation from normal. Kelly cannot be considered at fault for complications outside her control.

Case study 3.2 Anna's home birth

Anna has chosen a home birth having had a previous caesarean section for failure to progress. During the labour, Kelly monitors the fetal heart every 15 minutes but fails to recognise a significant reduction in the baseline fetal heart rate. She attributes the decelerations in the fetal heart following contractions to the fact that Anna is in the transitional stage of labour. Some time later, Kelly recognises a prolonged bradycardia and arranges for Anna to be transferred to the consultant unit. On arrival at the unit, 30 minutes later, Anna is taken to theatre for an emergency caesarean section. The baby requires extensive resuscitation and his prognosis is poor. Prior to attending Anna in labour, Kelly has not attended her regular fetal monitoring update, neither has she attended a recent emergency skills update.

In Case study 3.2, Kelly has failed to recognise signs of fetal compromise – particularly significant in a woman with a uterine scar. As a result she failed to seek emergency attention in a timely and appropriate manner. Furthermore, she has failed to keep up to date with requisite skills. Kelly could be held accountable for her omissions and/or failure to provide a reasonably expected standard of care.

In most cases, employers will accept vicarious liability for their employees. This means that the law will hold an institution liable for the actions of another (Jones and Jenkins, 2003). This position has arisen as a result of public policy, which recognises that organisations are in a much better position than their employees to compensate successful negligence claims. Whilst the defendant would be the NHS trust, the midwife would still be required to provide statements and possibly to give evidence in court. Independent midwives are not covered by vicarious liability unless they hold an honorary contract with a trust.

Preparing to support women who choose a controversial home birth

Whilst negligence cases are relatively few, there is much anecdotal evidence to suggest that midwives experience real anxiety and concern when supporting women who make controversial choices regarding place of birth. These anxieties no doubt arise from the personal and professional dilemmas that are heavily influenced by the culture in which midwives practise, as well as by our own personal values and beliefs.

The named community midwife may need the assistance of her SoM or manager to implement an individual package of care for a woman choosing controversial home birth. This choice often proves to be extremely contentious in a climate where individualised care is the gold standard of quality but rarely a reality in current service provision. Sadly, some professionals view the provision of targeted care in such cases as pandering to the wishes of difficult women in order to ensure they do not complain or give birth alone, but an agreed plan of care does ensure that midwives and women feel supported. It also ensures that the provision of midwifery care in labour remains consistent with statutory regulations and guidance.

It is vital that the midwife builds a relationship with the woman based on trust. In an emergency situation a woman is far more likely to value and respond to the professional judgement of the midwife if their relationship is based on mutual respect and honest, open dialogue. Continuity of carer is extremely important and every effort should be made to ensure that the woman is familiar with the midwives who are likely to be supporting her during her labour. The majority of NHS trusts will have a policy specifying the attendance of two midwives at all home births. If this is not the case, the attendance of two midwives should be positively considered if the midwife assesses that there is a degree of risk.

Early discussion with the woman regarding place of birth will allow the midwife to identify and acknowledge any gaps or deficiencies in her own practice (for instance updating on emergency drills). An SoM can assist in facilitating access to training as appropriate. Regular planned discussion sessions with an SoM will enable 'time out' for the community midwife to discuss any concerns and to make sure that he or she has access to effective support.

Legal advice is almost always readily available through NHS trust legal departments. Some organisations and legal departments will, however, often operate from what they consider to be a very proactive position that can appear to be very defensive from the woman's perspective. This clearly has the potential to lead to conflict, resulting in the woman becoming isolated from midwifery care. Legal teams may even become involved in direct communication with women on behalf of a trust. The rationale for this stance might be underpinned by a belief that formal legal communication will distance the professional from the decisions made by women, so that the midwife will not be seen to condone or support those choices which are viewed as contentious or which potentially predispose the woman to an adverse outcome. This approach can cause irreparable conflict between the woman and the midwife. There is a balance to be struck here and the midwife will need to be extremely sensitive in her approach. In exercising her statutory obligations, the midwife must be mindful that she must advocate for the woman regardless of her own beliefs and views.

Summary

Providers of care have an obligation to respond to government plans which call for the provision of choice regarding place of birth. This calls for home birth to form part of any maternity service provision. Whilst rare, the occasions when women choose to give birth at home, contrary to professional advice, can be fraught with anxiety for both professionals and the woman herself. It is crucial that the woman is given impartial, evidence-based information to facilitate informed decisions relating to her care.

Whatever the views held by professionals with regard to the woman's choice of birth environment, it is incumbent upon midwives to ensure that women continue to be provided with support and care. This is regardless of personal views and is supported and reiterated within statutory rules regulating the midwifery profession.

In formulating plans for the care of women who make what are deemed to be controversial choices, midwives can and should access a number of sources of support. These include SoMs, midwifery managers, NHS trust legal departments, the RCM and the NMC.

⚷ Key points

- Trusts have an obligation – but are not statutorily required – to provide services which allow women to exercise choice regarding place of birth.
- It is vital that women are given clear, unbiased, evidence-based information with which to inform their decision-making process.
- Early access to an SoM will ensure that the midwife receives help in providing ongoing support to women who choose controversial home birth.
- Clearly documented plans of care must be agreed between all parties in order to ensure that both the woman and the midwife feel informed and supported.
- Midwives have an obligation to provide care for women regardless of their choice of place of birth, providing that the trust that employs them provides this service.

References

Bolam vs Friern Hospital Management Committee (1957) 1WLR 582.

Campbell, R. and MacFarlane, A. (1994) *Where to be Born: The Debate and the Evidence*, 2nd edn. National Perinatal Epidemiology Unit, Oxford.

Carter, J. (2004) Working with women who make controversial choices about their care. The midwives' role and responsibility: can the regulatory framework help? www.nmc.uk.org (accessed on November 2006).

Davis, K. (1994) Responsibilities of choice . . . professionals must relinquish control of knowledge and become partners in the decision-making process. *Nursing Standard*, **8** (44), 20–21.

DH (2001) *Reference Guide to Consent for Examination and Treatment*. Department of Health, London.

DH (1993) *Changing Childbirth – The Report of the Expert Maternity Committee*. HMSO, London.

DH (2004) *The National Service Framework for Children, Young People and Maternity Services*. Department of Health, London.

Dimond, B. (2006) *Legal Aspects of Midwifery*, 3rd edn. Books for Midwives Press, London.

Fielder, A., Kirkham, M., Baker, K. and Sherridan, A. (2004) Trapped by thinking in opposites? *Midwifery Matters*, Issue 102, 6–9.

Flint, C. (2004) Maternity hospitals and suspensions. *British Journal of Midwifery*, **12**, 558.

Gill, R. and Stirratt, G. (2003) RCOG Ethics Committee Position Paper 2: November 2002. Patient and doctor autonomy within obstetrics and gynaecology. www.rcog.org.uk (accessed November 2006).

Gillon, R. (1986) *Philosophical Medical Ethics*, John Wiley, Chichester.

Great Britain (2005) *Mental Capacity Act 2005*, HMSO, London.

Great Britain (1977) *National Health Service Act 1977 (c49)*, HMSO, London.

House of Commons Health Committee (2003) *Choice in Maternity Services. Ninth Report of Session 2002–2003*, Volume 1. The Stationary Office, London.

Illich, I. (2001) *Limits to Medicine. Medical Nemesis: The Expropriation of Health*. Marion Boyars Publishers, London.

Jones, S. and Jenkins, R. (2003) *Law and the Midwife*, 2nd edn. Blackwell Science, Oxford.

Kirkham, M. and Stapleton, H. (2004) The culture of maternity services as a barrier to informed choice. In: *Informed Choice in Maternity Care* (ed. M. Kirkham). MacMillan Press, London.

Kirkham, M., Stapleton, H., Curtis, P. and Thomas, G. (2002) The inverse care law in antenatal care. *British Journal of Midwifery*, **10** (8), 509–513.

Levy, V. (2004) How midwives used protective steering to facilitate informed choice in pregnancy. In: *Informed Choice in Maternity Care* (ed. M. Kirkham). MacMillan Press, London.

Lewis, G. (2004) *Why Mothers Die 2000–2002: Report on Confidential Enquiry into Maternal Deaths in the UK*. RCOG Press, London.

Ley (1988) cited in Wilson, J. and Symon, A. (2002) *Clinical Risk Management in Midwifery: The Right to a Perfect Baby*. Books for Midwives Press, Oxford.

Magill-Cuerden, J. (2005) Report of issues arising form a review to support recommendations for guidance for home births. www.nmc.uk.org (accessed November 2006).

NICE (2006) (Draft 23 June 2006–29 August 2006) Intrapartum care: care of healthy women and their babies during childbirth. www.nice.org.uk (accessed March 2007).

NMC (2004a) *The NMC Code of Professional Conduct: Standards for Conduct, Performance and Ethics*. Nursing and Midwifery Council, London.

NMC (2004b) *Midwives' Rules and Standards*. Nursing and Midwifery Council, London.

NMC (2005) *Guidelines for Records and Record Keeping*. Nursing and Midwifery Council, London.

NMC (2006) NMC circular: midwives and home birth. www.nmc.uk.org (accessed November 2006).

Nolan, M. (2002) The consumer view. In: *Clinical Risk Management in Midwifery: The Right to a Perfect Baby* (eds J. Wilson and A. Symon). Books for Midwives Press, Oxford.

RCM (2001) Position Paper No 4a. Woman Centred Care www.rcm.org.uk (accessed September 2006).

RCM (2002) Position paper 25: home birth. *RCM Midwives Journal*, **5** (1), 26–29.

Rosser, J. (1998), Home birth: where does the buck stop? *Practising Midwife*, **1** (12), 4–5.

Sidaway vs. Bethlem Royal Hospital Governors (1985).

Walsh, D. (2006) *Risk and Normality in Maternity Care: Re-visioning the Risk for Normal Childbirth* (unpublished).

Wilson, J. and Symon, A. (2002) *Clinical Risk Management in Midwifery : the Right to a Perfect Baby?* Books for Midwives Press, Oxford.

Physiological third stage of labour and birth at home

Susan Blackburn

Within the midwifery profession, there is a noticeable groundswell of movement away from the medical model of childbirth towards normal, natural birth (Walsh, 2003; DH, 2004; RCM, 2005). An increase in the number of home births has been noted in many areas and many midwives openly pride themselves on understanding and facilitating an intervention-free birth in this environment. However, this understanding does not always extend to the final stage of the birth continuum – the birth of the placenta. This is very much an area where the medical model of care intervenes with the presumption that it can improve on nature.

This chapter seeks to illustrate a model of care that repositions midwifery practice during the third stage of labour in the home environment: placing it in a holistic, natural model of care that many women giving birth at home will choose. A review of the literature regarding the third stage and birth at home will ensure that practice suggestions are evidence based where possible. The physiology of the third stage will be described and a care pathway suggested that uses this knowledge to support midwifery practice in the absence of robust evidence. The likelihood of a safe and enjoyable third stage for all parties should then be enhanced.

Case study 4.1 illustrates a care pattern frequently offered to women who choose birth at home.

Case study 4.1 Care pattern at home birth

In the warm and cosy surroundings of Jane's bedroom, a natural labour ends in the birth of a well baby, born into her mother's hands and now enjoying skin-to-skin contact at the breast. The low, gentle music that accompanied the birth continues, and Jane and her husband are reclining on their own bed, gazing in wonder at their child. Peace fills the room as the new baby slowly becomes aware and establishes a regular breathing pattern. At this point an alert and focused midwife interjects, 'Did you want the injection to help deliver your afterbirth?'

Jane stops bonding with her newborn to look up at the midwife and consider the question. 'What is that?'

'It's a little injection that reduces blood loss and speeds up the delivery of your placenta. Did you have it with your last baby?'

Jane: 'I think so.'

Midwife: 'So you're happy to have it again?'

Jane, looking down at her infant again and murmurs 'Yes, if you think it's best.'

The midwife turns the baby over to clamp the cord and the father cuts it. The injection is given and Jane's thigh burns as if she has been stung. This soon fades and she continues to look at her baby. The midwife focuses on the cord and, after a few seconds, places a hand on Jane's lower abdomen to 'guard the uterus', firmly pushes down and commences controlled cord traction. Meanwhile, Jane has started to shake, and she feels cold and nauseous. She asks her husband to take the baby as a large contraction pains her. The baby startles and begins to cry as she is removed from her mother's breast to be wrapped and then soothed by her father. The midwife remains focused on the cord and pulls firmly. The placenta is delivered as Jane vomits and lies back with her eyes closed, wishing she did not feel so shaky and nauseous – she doesn't want to hold her baby at the moment.

Dad asks the midwife what is wrong with his wife. The midwife replies 'Oh, it's the side effect of the injection. Lots of women feel a bit sick and get the shakes – it'll go in a few minutes.' Dad cuddles his daughter and looks at his wife, who smiles back wanly.

Is there anything wrong with the care given in this scenario? Mother and baby are well and a beautiful home birth has been facilitated by a skilled midwife. What does it matter if the third stage wasn't entirely natural? From the woman's point of view, she may never think about that final stage of labour again. The baby is well, tended by her father, having suffered no obvious ill effects. From the midwife's point of view, she has carried out her routine practice competently, actively managing the third stage of labour and in so doing, possibly saving Jane from a life-threatening haemorrhage.

Anecdotal evidence suggests this is a common scenario at home births in the UK. Jane has had a lovely home birth but a more analytical approach might question whether the care outlined supported normal birth, gave the woman an informed choice or resulted in good outcomes for mother and baby.

Defining the midwife's role in the third stage of labour

Commonly, the third stage of labour is defined as the period from the delivery of the baby to the expulsion of the placenta and membranes, and control of bleeding (Morrin, 1999). The pervading view is that this is a 'dangerous' or 'hazardous' time (Morrin, 1999; Enkin et al., 2000). This view is supported by statistics in the UK showing postpartum haemorrhage (PPH) to be a leading cause of maternal death (Lewis, 2004). Midwives, who have been trained and immersed in a technological, medically managed and risk-obsessed birth environment, can view the third stage of labour as a fraught time, laden with danger. Training stresses the dangers, rehearses the emergency procedures and covers the elements of active management of third stage in detail. It is evident that some practitioners caring for women who choose physiological third stage do not consistently support natural physiology to its fullest extent, limiting and possibly reducing the safety of the third stage (Odent, 1998; Prendiville et al., 2000; Wagner, 2000).

A midwife's role in facilitating a natural physiological third stage of labour at home cannot simply be to sit back and wait. She or he must ensure that everything possible is done to support the normal physiology of birth, and the effects of normal physiology on the woman's and baby's experience must also be considered. A truly physiological third stage of labour is not a passive event. It involves active antenatal preparation, committed midwifery care during labour to support natural birth and avoid detrimental interventions, and diligent midwifery observations of the progress of the natural processes involved. A physiological approach to the third stage does not mean that care is not active – drugs and a hands-on approach are instead replaced by psychological and environmental elements, which actively promote normal physiological birth.

The physiology of the third stage of labour

The first step to ensuring a safe physiological third stage at home is to review and understand the underpinning physiology and the factors that affect its function.

Separation of the placenta

The birth hormones oxytocin, beta-endorphins, adrenalin, noradrenalin and prolactin are all secreted by the most primitive part of the human brain, the limbic cortex, and directly influence each other in a complicated 'hormonal dance' (Ockenden, 2001).

All three stages of labour are dependent on adequate secretion of the hormone oxytocin from the posterior lobe of the pituitary gland. This gland anticipates the heavy demand for oxytocin in labour by doubling in size during pregnancy as it lays down central stores of this hormone (Blackburn, 2003). Uterine muscle fibres are naturally contractile but activation of a contraction depends upon a complicated synergy of neurogenic systems. Oxytocin plays a major part in this process because it initiates the release of intracellular calcium. This supports complex cellular mechanisms that make uterine muscle fibres contract in harmony. It has been identified that high levels of adrenaline will suppress oxytocin production and release (Blackburn, 2003). The birth environment therefore has the potential to promote or inhibit contraction of the uterus, whatever the stage of labour. Odent (1998) places particular emphasis upon keeping the woman and the room warm during the third stage of labour to avoid an increase in adrenaline levels due to cold stress. Catecholamine concentrations peak as the baby is born and then return to normal levels within 2–20 minutes (Box 4.1).

Box 4.1 Practice point

- The midwife's role in maintaining an optimum environment for the constant production of oxytocin must extend throughout and beyond the birth of the placenta, to ensure a successful outcome (Odent, 1998).
- Odent (1994) goes further to suggest that all women who give birth in hospital surroundings should choose active management of the third stage because of the adverse effects of an unfamiliar setting upon adrenaline and oxytocin levels.

After the birth of the baby the volume of the uterus decreases rapidly, shearing the placenta from the uterine wall as the surface area of the placental bed diminishes in size (Morrin, 1999). Endogenous oxytocin ensures that contractions continue to retract the uterine muscle fibres. If the woman is left undisturbed, catecholamine levels fall, maternal oxytocin levels remain high, high levels of prolactin are released and the woman is physiologically stimulated to love and nurse her baby (Odent, 2002). Bleeding from torn blood vessels at the placental site is minimised as the contracted uterine muscles act as a living ligature.

Simultaneously, the physiological increase in clotting factors during pregnancy initiates coagulation and there is a further transient rise in these levels in response to the local trauma of separation. This dual physiological approach effectively prevents excessive blood loss from approximately 100 severed spiral arteries in the placental bed (Bates, 2002).

Separation of the placenta and neonatal transition

The newborn whose cord remains intact begins to establish regular breathing. Fetal blood within the placenta will continue to be oxygenated and circulate via the umbilical cord to the baby as long as the placenta remains attached to the uterine wall. The circulatory system changes from fetal to neonatal as the lungs perfuse. The foramen ovale closes and the ductus arteriosus begins to shut down in response to a number of physiological triggers. It is estimated that the lungs of a term baby of average size require approximately 45 ml of blood to expand the pulmonary vascular bed. The placenta and umbilical cord are estimated to contain 125–150 ml of fetal blood. It has been reported that a baby will receive a placental transfusion of approximately 80 ml within a few minutes of birth if positioned at the level of the mother's introitus (Yao and Lind, 1969). Christensen (2000) states that gravity facilitates the flow of blood from the placenta to the neonate, asserting that effective placental transfusion will occur within 3 minutes if the baby is held at or below the level of the placenta. As long as the cord is pulsating, and the baby positioned appropriately, she or he will be able to receive a physiologically regulated proportion of the placental/umbilical blood volume (Morrin, 1999; Frye, 2004).

Gaseous exchange is established gradually as the lungs expand; the baby relies on oxygenated cord blood during this time. Frye (2004) notes that even when the cord appears to be limp and without noticeable pulsation at birth (e.g. following cord compression during shoulder dystocia), a 'jump start effect' can occur a few seconds after birth and the cord will begin to pulsate again. The neonate then begins to respond as the placental circulation is re-established to increase her or his circulating blood volume.

As breathing becomes established the cord will stop pulsating. If the cord remains intact until no pulse is felt at the umbilicus and the baby is breathing regularly, the baby can be presumed to have regulated its blood volume. Once the transition from fetal to neonatal circulation is complete, there will be no further blood flow through the umbilical cord. The cord severed after this time, at least 10–12 cm from the baby's abdomen, will not bleed (Dunn, 1984). The blood within it will clot and seal the cord vessels.

Review of the evidence for physiological third stage of labour

It has been suggested that midwifery skills and the knowledge that will support a physiological third stage are lacking in practice because birth has moved into the medical, hospital-based arena (Harris, 2001). It is indeed possible for a midwife to train and practise without ever seeing or facilitating a physiological third stage of labour (Walsh, 2003). The fundamental role of the midwife, however, is to fully support normal, natural pregnancy and birth, in any environment, to include the care of women choosing physiological third stage at home (NMC, 2004a; Thewlis, 2006).

The information that midwives offer should be evidence based, enabling women to make an informed choice regarding their care.

Following an extensive search of the literature and pertinent databases (using the key words third stage management, postpartum haemorrhage, active management, physiological third stage and home birth), no formal research in the form of randomised controlled trials was identified to compare the benefits of actively managed and physiological third stage in the home birth environment. All such assessments have taken place in a hospital setting under less than natural circumstances where true physiological birth is not supported well and interventions in normal birth are common (Anderson, 2002).

Studies included in the much quoted Cochrane review *Active versus expectant management in the third stage of labour* (Prendiville et al., 2000) did not exclude women with risk factors and other labour interventions which predispose to PPH. These factors will rarely be encountered in the home birth setting, where the vast majority of women are designated at low risk for PPH. Indeed, the review states that 'Active management should be the routine management of choice for women expecting to deliver a baby by vaginal delivery in a maternity hospital'. It goes on to say that 'the implications are less clear for other settings, including domiciliary practice'.

No study was identified in the literature review that examined the benefits and risks to the term newborn of third stage management methods, as a primary outcome. In contrast, detailed study of the physiology of the third stage and its importance to the newborn's transition to extra-uterine life has been carried out and it is widely acknowledged that early cord clamping deprives the neonate of blood volume (Mercer and Skovgaard, 2004; Cernadas et al., 2005). The long-term effects of early cord clamping have not been studied, but Chapparo et al.'s (2006) randomised controlled trial of Mexican infants clearly demonstrated a beneficial effect on iron levels at 6 months of age when cord clamping was delayed for 2 minutes.

A physiological third stage will enable full transfusion of the placental–fetal blood to the newborn, providing it with up to 30% greater blood volume and hence 30% greater red blood cell volumes. This enables the newborn to cope with temperature reduction at birth, more oxygenated red cells being available to support the increased metabolic rate resulting from cold stress (Frye, 2004; Mercer and Skovgaard, 2004).

Research has suggested that one of the biggest causes of feto–maternal blood transfusion may be actively managed third stage (Wickham, 2001). It is proposed that a physiological third stage reduces the likelihood of feto–maternal transfusion occurring by removing traumatic causes. These are suggested as the sudden tearing of the placenta resulting from controlled cord traction, forcing fetal blood into maternal tissues when 'guarding' the uterus and preventing adequate maternal blood loss from the placental site to cleanse fetal blood out of the mothers system via the birth canal, through early clamping of the umbilical cord. A literature review by Soltani et al. (2005) found that more evidence is needed to ascertain the validity of these proposals but the theoretical potential for harm must be recognised. In line with ethical principles and as stated in the NMC *Code of Professional Conduct* 'any intervention to the birth process should have clear benefit for either mother or baby and the benefit should outweigh the risks of the intervention' (NMC, 2004b).

It can thus be argued that a clear lack of evidence to support interventions in the home birth environment indicates that a midwife's default practice should support physiological third stage until circumstances arise which necessitate further intervention. This is a view supported by the RCM, who state that 'Physiological management can be seen as the logical ending to a normal physiological labour' (RCM, 2005). Many midwives will be extremely nervous of taking this expectant approach to the third stage of labour, so ingrained is the fear of haemorrhage and so limited the experience of natural birth at home. A brief review of the facts behind the most commonly quoted reasons for intervention may alleviate some of these concerns and facilitate discussion with women as they plan their care.

The third stage and maternal mortality and morbidity

The incidence of PPH resulting in maternal death in the UK is 6.7 per million and the rate has been seen to double since the previous triennial report (Lewis, 2004). Reasons for this may include a rise in the number of women at high risk of PPH and, in many cases of maternal death, substandard professional care was found to have contributed significantly to this devastating outcome. None of the women who died had a planned home birth.

No evidence was found which assessed the mother's physical experience of the effect of blood loss. The key outcome measured in all studies is volume of loss rather than a measure of the effect of that loss upon women's health. The Independent Midwifery Association (whose clients' birth predominantly at home and over 60% of whom have a normal birth and physiological third stage) carried out an audit of clients' health outcomes (Milan, 2005). This illustrated the fact that although a higher than average incidence of PPH, defined as greater than 500 ml estimated blood loss, was noted at birth, only one woman had an associated problem at discharge, which may or may not have been linked to the amount of third stage blood loss. It has also been observed that whilst immediate post-birth blood loss is noted to be higher with physiological third stage, blood loss appears to continue for a longer period of time in the puerperium following an actively managed third stage (Wickham, 2000).

Two problems arise from the focus on volume of blood loss rather than effect. Firstly, it is now recognised that blood loss is not easily measured and is frequently underestimated for the vast majority of women (Edwards, 1999; Frye, 2004). Secondly, the physiological effect of blood loss is unique to the individual. A 200 ml blood loss can cause symptomatic anaemia in a small woman with low antenatal haemoglobin levels, whilst a 1000 ml loss can leave another woman with no symptoms at all. It has been argued that, due to the 30% or greater increase in blood volume over the pregnancy, a well woman with normal haemoglobin levels who experiences a PPH following a term birth can withstand a blood loss of 1000 ml before feeling an effect (Edwards, 1999; Frye, 2004). As Wickham (2001) points out, 500 ml is only slightly more than the average amount of blood that a donor gives at a session, after which a cup of tea and 10-minute sit down is deemed sufficient therapy.

Duration of the third stage of labour

There is no good quality evidence that supports the premise that a physiological third stage at home will take longer than one that is actively managed. Observation suggests that in a well-supported, truly physiological birth the placenta will be birthed within minutes of the baby (Odent, 1998). Botha's (1968) classic study identified that the mean length of the third stage was 3.5 minutes when the placental end of the cord was left unclamped.

The origins of the imposition of time limits on the third stage of labour are difficult to ascertain. Coombs and Laros (1991) and Dombrowski et al. (1995) both identified a significant increase in PPH in the 30–60 minute window following the birth of the baby. Optimum outcomes in these large studies were associated with the placenta being birthed in the first 30 minutes. A longer duration can be an indication of a problem such as an adherent placenta and the skilled midwife will recognise the need for transfer to hospital and appropriate obstetric intervention. It is possible, however, for a midwife unaccustomed to supporting physiological third stage to overlook the physiological cues indicating that the placenta has in fact separated and is ready to be birthed. In these cases, allowing time, good emotional support and the skills of a confident midwife will facilitate the physiological birth of the placenta.

The time limits imposed by systems of care provision and issues such as understaffing should not impact upon the well-being and choices of an individual. Over-stretched maternity services have created pressures that demand the freeing up of labour ward beds as quickly as possible. Whilst this will not happen at a home birth, the midwife may still be due to attend a clinic and half a dozen or more home visits after attending a birth at home and will be under pressure of a demanding workload. However, under the ethical premise that care should do no harm, intervening with active management for these reasons cannot be justified.

Antenatal preparation for the third stage of labour

If a physiological third stage is to be as safe as possible then care and preparation should start in the antenatal period. It is apparent that most women (especially those expecting their first baby) know little of the choices open to them in relation to the third stage and a brief discussion in the second stage of labour is inadequate and highly inappropriate.

Good midwifery antenatal care allows women the opportunity to explore their options for management of the third stage of labour. Community midwives can do much to dispel myths and allay any fears through provision of evidence-based information, supported by accurate physiological facts.

Information giving and informed choice

There is evidence to suggest that women do not choose their preferred method of third stage management but, instead, are directed to whichever method the midwife advises or prefers. Harris' (2001) exploration of midwifery practice in the third stage of labour and Edwards' (2000) survey of women's experience of home birth both revealed that many women are not choosing the method of third stage management. They are generally directed towards active management by midwives working in a risk-averse culture, in an environment which favours interventionist practice. Women who have experienced both pharmacologically and physiologically managed third stages demonstrated a preference for the empowering experience of a physiological birth of the placenta (Jill, 2005; Gascoigne, personal communication).

Trials comparing active versus physiological management in a hospital setting (Prendiville et al., 2000) indicate either no preference on the mother's part, or a preference for active management due to a perceived shortening of duration of third stage recommending this model of care. When one considers the hospital as a birth setting it is perhaps no surprise that this intervention, despite its associated side effects, might be preferred. A stark hospital environment, lack of privacy and often a lack of overall control of the birth process does not enable a woman to safely and contentedly await the arrival of the placenta. It is arguable that women choosing to give birth in a home setting will be more likely to await the natural birth of the placenta, simply because they are able to feel comfortable and relaxed and have the luxury of enjoying the privacy of their own surroundings.

The information offered by midwives must, of course, be balanced. When discussing active management in relation to birth at home it should be presented as an option but is possible to say that there is no specific evidence to support this intervention in low-risk women. Active management, in itself, is associated with a number of risks and significant drug-related side effects. A woman should be made aware of these in order to make a fully informed choice.

Antenatal identification and exploration of the implications of risk factors for complicated third stage will also help women make an informed choice about the management of their third stage of labour (Box 4.2).

Box 4.2 Risk factors for complicated third stage

- Placenta accreta/percreta
- Previous caesarean section
- Previous retained placenta
- Pre-existing clotting disorders
- Multiple pregnancy
- Pre-eclampsia
- Traumatic birth, e.g. shoulder dystocia
- Full bladder
- Abnormal first and second stage of labour
- Use of pharmacological pain relief in labour

Frye (2004)

There is a commonly held belief that pre-existing anaemia is a risk factor for PPH. Whilst it is not a cause of bleeding, if present at the onset of labour it can be detrimental to the ability of the woman both to labour efficiently and to cope with blood loss following the birth (Page, 2000). Improving diet to focus on ways to increase the intake of natural iron, and supplementation with ferrous sulphate where indicated, can treat anaemia and reduce the risk of adverse effects of blood loss.

Ultimately, the decision about care in the third stage is the woman's, although it is worth noting that whilst a woman may decline an intervention, she may not insist that a midwife carry out an intervention inappropriately. Sometimes, women who have a number of risk factors will choose a natural home birth against advice and opt for a physiological approach for the birth of the placenta despite the recommendations outlined in current guidelines. Some, however, will weigh risk differently and will opt for active management. Others may change their minds about a physiological third stage half-way through their labour or at the last minute, perhaps because they are tired of waiting and want to shower or sleep.

With good planning and documentation, all elements of the birth of the placenta can be discussed antenatally so that whoever attends the birth can act appropriately, according to the woman's informed choice.

Planning a safe birthing environment at home

Part of the midwife's role is to help a woman create a safe, warm and private birthing environment to support an efficient labour and birth and to maintain this environment until the birth of the placenta is safely completed. It cannot be taken for granted that women choosing to birth at home will instinctively act to make that environment as safe as possible. It is possible that social conditioning and modern customs have subjugated these instincts. Women may subconsciously conform to the norm of labouring and birthing confined to the bedroom, worrying about their anxious partners, their children, the neighbours and even the carpet. Midwives can encourage women to explore how they might act instinctively, consider who should be present at the birth and make arrangements for childcare (or support for children who wish be present for the birth of their new sibling). It is also important to discuss how to manage birth partners or other people who are distracting and causing anxiety. Discuss what activities, music, smells and places increase the woman's sense of well-being and relaxation. Whilst we know that low lights and quiet privacy will generally engender a calm, relaxed atmosphere, it is possible that some women will feel most relaxed within a noisier and busier atmosphere in the presence of a number of family or friends.

Midwifery practice to support physiological third stage of labour

At all times during the third stage of labour, the midwife should remain calmly observant of the physical reactions and adjustment of both mother and baby (see Table 4.1). Maintaining a calm and warm environment will maximise the woman's oxytocin production but the

Table 4.1 Continuum of events and activities around the third stage: woman's, baby's and midwife's experiences.

	Mother	Placenta and cord	Baby	Midwife
Birth	Uterine volume rapidly reduced Adrenaline production decreases Oxytocin production continues Beta-endorphin production continues Picks up baby/baby placed skin to skin	Placenta attached and perfused Cord pulsating	Skin to skin with mother Dried as needed Pressure and temperature stimulation Lungs begin to perfuse with blood Transition to neonatal circulation begins	Acts calmly to promote maternal oxytocin production and decrease maternal adrenaline production Passes baby to mother Assists mother and father to dry baby Places baby skin to skin on mother's abdomen
1 to 2 minutes	Begins to return to conscious awareness May not be absorbed with baby as adjusting to feelings of ending of birth Uterus not contracting but smaller Oxytocin production continues Endorphin production continues	Placenta attached but starting to separate Cord pulsating	Remains skin to skin Begins to breathe air Transition to neonatal circulation continues	Acts calmly Monitors blood loss and signs of maternal compromise Watches baby for signs of adaptation Helps mother to comfortable position on clean 'inco' pad
3 to 5 minutes	Focused on baby – skin to skin Uterus begins to contract and retract May become distressed as contractions begin Clotting begins at the placental site Some maternal blood loss noted per vaginam	Placenta shears off uterine wall and descends to lower uterine segment Cord pulsating at neonatal end	Breathing regulates	Reassures mother that contractions are natural and good. Birth nearly finished Ensures calm quiet warm atmosphere Ensures baby breathing regularly Skin to skin contact maintained Monitors blood loss and signs of maternal compromise
5 to 30 minutes	Feels contraction and bulk of placenta descend into birth canal Trickle of maternal blood per vaginam continues Woman may feel urge to push placenta out	Cord lengthens Placenta descends into the vagina No pulsation palpable along length of cord	Baby breathing Blood volume is stable Transition to neonatal circulation achieved Baby put to breast and may suckle	Reassures mother to do as she feels Maintains calm quiet warm atmosphere Monitors blood loss and signs of maternal compromise

midwife must always be ready to offer reassurance and, if necessary, initiate appropriate intervention. Once the baby is born, it is often expected that he or she should immediately be washed, weighed and handed round for all to admire, amidst bright lights and lively conversation. It is important for birth supporters to appreciate the importance of the environment and immediate, prolonged skin-to-skin contact between the woman and her baby, in order to facilitate the 'hormonal dance' vital for an effective third stage. Breastfeeding is a key catalyst for stimulation of the post-birth flood of oxytocin necessary for safe physiological third stage. If the woman does not intend to breastfeed at all she should still be encouraged to consider skin-to-skin contact in the initial post-birth period. Covering the woman and baby with warm towels or blankets will enable them to enjoy skin-to-skin contact and the benefit of neonatal temperature regulation. Manual nipple stimulation is known to facilitate oxytocin production (Enkin et al., 2000). This is a theoretical alternative to the oxytocin producing effect of breastfeeding but it is also a very intimate act. Few women would feel relaxed enough to perform this intervention effectively in the presence of a midwife and a number of birth supporters.

Observation suggests that in the immediate post-birth period women are tense and adrenaline fuelled but this subsides after a few moments and many women are overwhelmed with the urge to lie down (Odent, 1998). The position preferred by the mother will best enhance her ability to relax with her baby and enable the normal physiological birth of the placenta. Resting on a comfortable mattress with clean dry 'inco' pads or towels will help her to feel relaxed. There is some evidence of a link between increased blood loss and upright positions during the third stage (Jahanfar et al., 2004). It is argued, however, that this may simply be a more immediate and visible loss of a normal volume of blood as the placenta separates, as it does not remain pooled in the uterus.

Separation and expulsion of the placenta

Mismanagement of the third stage of labour is the most likely cause of PPH (Odent, 1998; Varney et al., 2004). Varney and colleagues propose a number of rules for good management in general but Box 4.3 illustrates important points for a physiological approach.

Box 4.3 Practice point

- Do not massage the uterus prior to placental separation
- Discipline yourself in the art of waiting – do not feel pressurised to interfere unwisely in a natural process
- Become an expert in diagnosing placental separation

Adapted from Varney et al. (2004: 907).

There are a number of signs to indicate that a placenta has separated. As it shears away from the uterine wall at the level of the spongy layer of the decidua the resulting blood loss collects as a retroplacental clot (Blackburn, 2003). The weight of this clot will encourage the placenta to descend into the lower segment of the uterus by the force of gravity. As this occurs there will be a visible trickle of blood per vaginam. This descent will also be indicated by a lengthening of the umbilical cord. If the midwife observes the woman's abdomen at this point it is possible to see that the uterus has changed its position and its shape. The soft, wide fundus remains about 2 cm below the navel until the uterus contracts and the placenta separates. It then becomes hard and round, rising to the level of the umbilicus. As the placenta is expelled, the uterus will contract and sink to 4 or 5 cm below the woman's umbilicus (Frye, 2004).

Odent (1998) is clear in his opinion that any intervention in the immediate post-birth period is unnecessary and detrimental. He advocates continued but unobtrusive observation of the woman and her baby and does not check for separation unless there is the rare event of a 1-hour delay. Separation can then be identified if the fingertips are used to gently press just above the woman's symphysis pubis and the cord does not move. If the placenta is still adherent the cord will retract a little, back up into the vagina, when pressure is exerted.

When the woman feels the placenta descend into the vagina she may need to be encouraged to bear down to birth the placenta. Many women will feel anxious at this point and need reassurance that although the contractions may be painful, the birth of the placenta will feel much easier than that of the baby – no bones! Some encouragement may be needed to expend a last bit of energy in pushing the placenta out, but many women push this amazing temporary organ out spontaneously as they identify the sensation of its descent into the vagina. The cord can then be clamped and cut.

Requests for 'lotus birth' are increasing in the UK according to anecdotal reports. A 'lotus birth' involves leaving the placenta and cord intact until natural separation occurs at around 3 to 10 days (Rachana, 2000). The placenta should be checked as usual and then washed, covered in salt and packed in the woman's chosen wrapping. Some women have placenta bags specially made.

For those choosing to separate the placenta from the baby immediately after the third stage is complete, it must be remembered that cultural significance may be attached to its fate. Some cultures consider it a part of the baby, requiring that it be buried near the family home (Anand, 2000; Davies, 2002). Most women will be happy for the midwife to dispose of the placenta via the hospital incineration system but it should be remembered that the placenta remains the property of the mother and its disposal should be discussed with her. For health and safety reasons the placenta should be transported from home to hospital in an appropriate container.

Assessing maternal blood loss

With an intact cord, any vaginal blood loss will be maternal in origin. As discussed previously, the measurement of blood loss is difficult and frequently inaccurate, but the effect of any blood loss on the mother's circulatory system must be observed closely. Routine monitoring of pulse and blood pressure, intrusive attempts to visualise vaginal blood loss and unnecessary checks for cessation of cord pulsation will interfere with the physiology of a natural third stage. These interventions will distract the woman to inhibit the flow of endorphins and oxytocin as she bonds with her baby. They should be avoided unless the woman's general condition, consciousness level, pallor or respiratory rate causes concern.

It must be emphasised that massaging the uterus prior to separation is unsafe practice. It can cause concealed retroplacental bleeding due to partial separation, causing the fundus to balloon as the uterus becomes tense and distended. If partial separation does occur, then symptomatic hypovolaemia will prompt urgent intervention. Call for help, apply bimanual compression, resuscitate the woman and transfer her to hospital as soon as possible to deliver the placenta manually. This nightmare scenario is largely avoidable if a midwife heeds Varney et al.'s (2004) advice to watch and wait. Use your skills of observation to assess the process of separation, rather than using your hands.

As the Independent Midwifery Association statistics evidence, women birthing at home will sometimes experience PPH and the emergency care in these cases will include administration of intramuscular or intravenous oxytocic drugs. Whilst in an emergency a midwife is permitted to take life-saving actions without consent, the antenatal discussion can include seeking permission and consent to give these drugs should an emergency situation arise. It is crucial that community midwives are competent to deal with obstetric emergencies in the home and regular updates are mandatory to maintain these skills.

Retained placenta

The majority of women will have birthed their placenta within 30 minutes of the birth of the baby. If there is no sign of this after 30–60 minutes, the mother can be encouraged to change position and empty her bladder. Palpating the bladder is inadvisable as this can interfere with the natural synchronisation of contractions and process of separation. Moving to a kneeling position will often apply enough gravitational and abdominal pressure to expel a separated placenta spontaneously.

The point at which the placenta is considered as retained is debateable. If the condition of the woman is stable, she may want to wait longer than the hour generally prescribed in current guidelines before agreeing to transfer into hospital. The option to attempt active management prior to transfer springs to mind but evidence to support this decision is limited. However, the NICE (2007) guideline for intrapartum care states that failure to deliver the placenta after 60 minutes indicates a need to change to active management. Long (2003) discusses 'adaptive' care in the third stage of labour to explore some situations where a physiological third stage is affected by unforeseen circumstances, but the examples offered relate to clamping and cutting of the cord rather than the scenario outlined above in a home setting. Adaptive care is defined as 'any care that involves a combination of components from "active" and "natural"'. Long (2003) quotes Chalmers et al. (1989) to identify that adaptive approaches are unevaluated and should therefore be viewed with a great degree of caution.

The increased risk of haemorrhage in these circumstances has to be considered, bearing in mind the threefold increase in incidence of PPH in the 30–60 minute window described by Coombs and Laros (1991). Data from a study of 45 000 women in the USA supported the findings of Coombs and Laros, and also indicated that 40% of women who have not birthed their placenta by 35 minutes after the birth of the baby will undergo manual removal (Dombrowski et al., 1995).

Monitoring the baby immediately post birth

If the umbilical cord remains intact and pulsating, the baby will still be partially oxygenated via the placental transfusion. As a result, he or she may well take longer to establish regular respirations than the infant whose cord is subjected to early clamping and cutting as a component of active management of the third stage. The mechanisms causing the baby to make the change from fetal to neonatal circulation include respiratory triggers in the medulla, a reduction in oxygen, accumulation of carbon dioxide and a drop in ambient temperature as the baby leaves the intra uterine environment (Sweet, 1999: 784).

This slower transition to extra-uterine life may be unfamiliar to the midwife who is used to actively managing the third stage, but an awareness of this natural adaptation is vital if the midwife is to gain confidence in supporting the overall process of physiological birth (Long, 2003).

During the moments following the birth of the baby, the midwife will assess the baby's colour, tone, heart rate and state of the umbilical cord. If resuscitative measures are needed immediately, these can be carried out with the cord still attached in all but the rarest of circumstances (Box 4.4).

Box 4.4 Practice point

- The intact cord provides a lifeline prior to the point of placental separation when neonatal resuscitation is required.
- Mercer et al. (2005) advocate lowering the infant with an intact cord below the level of the perineum and 'milking' of the cord to support resuscitative efforts in infants whose heart rate is less than 100 beats per minute.

In the rare event that the cord snaps, the baby's end should be clamped and close monitoring will be essential as the infant may have lost blood volume. It is not necessary to clamp the maternal end of the cord. Doing so will interfere further with the physiology of the third stage.

When the third stage is complete, in most cases enough fetal blood remains within the large vessels of the placenta to enable cord blood sampling where women have a rhesus negative blood group. Anecdotally, some midwives do take blood successfully from the cord prior to the birth of the placenta without undue blood loss. However, this practice is unresearched and could theoretically compromise placental transfusion if the puncture site oozes.

Water birth and physiological third stage

There has been much debate surrounding the issue of best practice in management of the third stage of labour when women choose to give birth in water in hospital and at home. The theoretical risk of water embolism has been used as a reason to ask women to leave the pool for the birth of the placenta. The inability to monitor blood loss is another.

There is no recorded case of water embolism to date and the author of the original article mentioning this theoretical risk has since commented that he regrets having raised the issue because it has been used to limit women's access to water during labour (Odent, 1983). Odent has further questioned the rationale underpinning the birth of a baby and completion of the third stage in water, stating that water is in fact an unnatural birth environment for most mammals and recognising that there is no research which comprehensively examines the effect of water immersion on third stage physiology.

Burns' (2001) audit, of more than 1000 women who chose to give birth in water, identified that there was no increase in the rate of PPH. More than half of these women had a physiological third stage. Visual assessment of blood loss is initially possible in clear water as the blood is seen to flow outwards from the mother. Whilst a rapid haemorrhage will certainly be noticeable within the water, a smaller but persistent bleed may not be, as the blood is dispersed and water darkens and clouds very quickly. Frye (2004) suggests placing a white towel under the mother in a dark-coloured pool in order to highlight vaginal blood loss.

Very close attention must be paid to the woman's physical state if she remains in the water for a physiological third stage. If the midwife suspects a haemorrhage, she or he should call for urgent assistance and remove the woman from the pool immediately in order to actively intervene.

Summary

It must be remembered that the midwife's primary duty of care is to her client. A woman's choices should not be limited by the model of care in which the midwife works. These models must be adaptable in order to provide women with information to underpin their decisions wherever possible. Independent midwives have the ability to arrange their work schedule with the utmost flexibility and can plan for a physiological third stage as the natural conclusion to an intervention-free birth, in partnership with the woman over a period of time. Community midwives might consider exploring new ways of working with their managers to enable them to improve continuity of care for those women who choose home birth.

There is no scientific evidence to recommend either active management with prophylactic oxytocin or physiological management of the third stage in the home birth environment but exploration of the physiology of natural birth in this chapter has supported a physiological approach. This comes with the proviso that a safe physiological third stage involves careful antenatal preparation and an informed approach to intrapartum care that supports natural birth within an optimal environment. Midwives have a duty of care to be competent in all aspects of third stage management. If a midwife feels that she or he has training needs to develop competence and confidence in caring for women who choose a physiological third stage, the support of a supervisor of midwives should be sought.

A calm, confident, skilled midwife is the key to safe physiological birth of the placenta at home.

⬤▭═⚷   **Key points**

- The available evidence comparing active and physiological management of the third stage of labour relates exclusively to birth in the hospital environment.
- Women should be offered information during their pregnancy to underpin an informed choice regarding their choice of third stage management in labour, whatever the location for the place of birth.
- Preparation for a safe and effective physiological third stage of labour at home should begin in the antenatal period, in partnership with the woman.
- When the birth of the placenta is delayed there is an increased incidence of postpartum haemorrhage during the 30–60 minute window.
- Hypovolaemic neonates will benefit from resuscitation supported by placental transfusion when the cord remains intact.
- Midwives have a professional responsibility to ensure their competence in all aspects of third stage management.

References

Anand, K. (2000) The placenta and cord in other cultures. In: *Lotus Birth* (ed. S. Rachana). Greenwood Press, Steels Creek, Australia.

Anderson, T. (2002) Out of the laboratory; back to the darkened room. *MIDIRS Midwifery Digest*, **12** (1), 68.

Bates, C. (ed.) (2002) *The Third Stage of Labour: RCM Brown Study Series*. Royal College of Midwives, London.

Blackburn, S.T. (2003) *Maternal, Fetal and Neonatal Physiology: A Clinical Perspective*, 2nd edn. Saunders, St. Louis.

Botha, M.C. (1968) The management of the umbilical cord in labour. *South African Journal of Obstetrics and Gynaecology*, **6**, 30–33.

Burns, E. (2001) Waterbirth. *MIDIRS Midwifery Digest*, **11**(Suppl. 2), S10–13.

Cernadas, J.M.C., Carroli, G., Pelligrini, L. et al. (2005) The effect of timing of cord clamping on neonatal venous hematocrit values and clinical outcome at term: a randomised controlled trial. *Pediatrics*, **117**, 779–786.

Chalmers, I., Enkin, M., Kierse, M. (1989) *Effective Care in Pregnancy and Childbirth*. Oxford University Press, Oxford.

Chaparro, C.M., Neufeld, L.M., Alavez, G.T., Cedillo, R.E., Dewey, K.G. (2006) Effect of timing of umbilical cord clamping on iron status in Mexican infants: a randomised controlled trial. *Lancet*, **367**, 1997–2004.

Christensen, R.D. (2000) *Hematologic Problems of the Neonate*. WB Saunders, Philadelphia.

Coombs, C.A. and Laros, R.K. (1991) Prolonged third stage of labour: morbidity and risk factors. *Obstetrics and Gynaecology*, **77**, 863–867.

Davies, R. (2002) The placenta: symbolic organ or waste product? *The Practising Midwife.* **5** (11), 19–21.

DH (2004) *National Service Framework for Children, Young People and Maternity Services: Maternity Services.* Department of Health, London.

Dombrowski, M.P., Bottoms, S.F., Saleh, A.A., Hurd, W.W., Romero, R. (1995) Third stage of labor: analysis of duration and clinical practice. *American Journal of Obstetrics and Gynecology,* **172**, 1279–1284.

Dunn, P.M. (1984) The third stage and fetal adaptation. In: *Perinatal Medicine. Proceedings of the IX European Congress of Perinatal Medicine held in Dublin* (eds. J. Clinch and T. Matthews). MTP Lancaster, Boston.

Edwards, N.P. (1999) *Delivering Your Placenta: The Third Stage.* Association for Improvements in Maternity Services.

Edwards, N.P. (2000) Women planning homebirths. In: *The Midwife–Mother Relationship* (ed. M. Kirkham). Palgrave Macmillan, Basingstoke.

Enkin, M., Keirse, M.J.N.C., Neilson, J. et al. (2000) *A Guide to Effective Care in Pregnancy and Childbirth,* 3rd edn. Oxford University Press, Oxford.

Frye, A. (2004) *Holistic Midwifery: (Volume 2) Care During Labour and Birth.* Labrys Press, Portland, Oregon.

Harris, T. (2001) Changing the focus for the third stage of labour. *British Journal of Midwifery,* **9** (1), 7–12.

Jahanfar, S., Amini, L., Jamshidi, R. (2004) Third and fourth stages of labour: sitting position. *British Journal of Midwifery,* **12** (7), 437.

Jill (2005) Experiences of third stage. *AIMS Journal,* **17** (4), 11.

Lewis, G (2004) *Why Mothers Die 2000–2002 – Report on Confidential Enquiries into Maternal Deaths in the United Kingdom.* RCOG Press, London.

Long, L. (2003) Defining third stage of labour care and discussing optimal practice. *MIDIRS Midwifery Digest,* **13** (3), 366–370.

Mercer, J.S. and Skovgaard, R.L. (2004) Fetal to neonatal transition: first, do no harm. In: *Normal Childbirth: Evidence and Debate* (ed. S. Downe), p. 141. Churchill Livingstone, Edinburgh.

Milan, M. (2005) Independent midwifery compared with other caseload practice. *MIDIRS Midwifery Digest,* **15** (4), 439–448.

Morrin, N.A. (1999) Midwifery care in the third stage of labour. In: *Mayes Midwifery* (ed. B. Sweet), 12th edn. Baillière Tindall, London.

NICE (2007) *Intrapartum Care: Care of women and their babies during childbirth.* National Institute for Health and Clinical Excellence, London.

NMC (2004a) *Midwives Rules and Standards.* Nursing and Midwifery Council, London.

NMC (2004b) *The NMC Code of Professional Conduct: Standards for Performance Conduct and Ethics.* Nursing and Midwifery Council, London.

Ockenden, J. (2001) The hormonal dance of labour: Can we teach women how to get 'in the mood' for labour? In: *Midwifery Best Practice Practice,* Vol. 2 (ed. Wickham). Books for Midwives, Edinburgh.

Odent, M. (1983) Birth under water. *Lancet,* **2** (8365–8366), 1476–1477.

Odent, M. (1994) *The Farmer and the Obstetrician.* Free Association Books, London.

Odent, M. (1998) Don't manage the third stage of labour! *The Practising Midwife*, **1** (9), 31–33.

Odent, M. (2002) The first hour following birth. *Midwifery Today*, **61** (Spring), 9–11.

Page, L.A. (2000) *The New Midwifery: Science and Sensitivity in Practice*. Churchill Livingstone, Edinburgh.

Prendiville, W.J., Elbourne, D., McDonald, S. (2000) Active versus expectant management in the third stage of labour. *Cochrane Database of Systematic Reviews*, Issue 3.

Rachana, S. (2000) *Lotus Birth*. Greenwood Press, Steels Creek, Australia.

RCM (2005) *Midwifery Practice Guideline: Evidence based Guidelines for Midwifery-led Care in Labour*, pp. 76–80. Royal College of Midwives, London.

Soltani, H., Dickinson, F., Leung, T.N. (2005) The effect of placental cord drainage in the third stage of labour on feto-maternal transfusion: a systematic review. *Evidence Based Midwifery*, **3** (2), 64–68.

Sweet, B. (1999) Physiology and care of the newborn. In: *Mayes' Midwifery* (ed. B. Sweet). 12th edn. Bailliere Tindall, London.

Thewlis, S. (2006) *Circular 8: Midwives and Home Birth*. Nursing and Midwifery Council, London.

Varney, H., Kriebs, J.M., Gegor, C.L. (2004) *Varney's Midwifery*, 4th edn. Jones and Bartlett, Massachusetts.

Wagner, M. (2000) *Fish Can't See Water: The Need to Humanize Birth in Australia*. Homebirth Australia Conference, Noosa. http://www.acegraphics.com.au/articles/wagner03.html (accessed 7.1.07).

Walsh, D. (2003) Haemorrhage and the third stage of labour. *British Journal of Midwifery*, **11** (2), 72.

Wickham, S. (2000) Further thoughts on the third stage. *MIDIRS Midwifery Digest*. **10** (2), 204–205.

Wickham, S. (2001) *Anti-D in Midwifery: Panacea or Paradox?* Books for Midwives, Oxford.

Yao, A.C. and Lind, J. (1969) Effect of gravity on placental transfusion. *Lancet*, **2**, 505.

Teaching antenatal classes: how can midwives deliver?

Ann Bradshaw

'Experiences that are multi-sensory, dramatic, unusual or emotionally strong are remembered for longer and in more detail than ordinary routine explanations' Ginnis (2004)

Teachers from any discipline are always eager to hear about new ideas that will enhance their teaching and make learning an enjoyable experience for their students. This chapter aims to give the reader a layperson's look at how adults learn, de-mystifying terms such as 'global aims' and 'learning outcomes'. It will offer some straightforward tips on how to put antenatal teaching sessions together and provide some examples of teaching ideas. Some of these have been passed on by word of mouth; some have come from books and been adapted. It is hoped that they will be of some help to those midwives who are struggling to find fresh ideas to increase their confidence in teaching. The knock-on effect should result in teaching sessions that are much more effective from a student's (or in this case, parent's) point of view.

As an advanced antenatal teacher for the National Childbirth Trust (NCT) for 15 years, and an associate lecturer for midwifery students, my passion for teaching grows almost daily. I know why I teach. I have my own underlying beliefs, which shine through in my teaching and my hope is that this becomes part of my clients' deeper learning experience.

Many midwives teach antenatal classes because they have to, not because they want to. There is no luxury of choice. Even so, all midwives will have deep-seated beliefs about why they are midwives and what drives them to do the job they do. As a midwife you are teaching during most of your working life. Every time you talk with a woman and her partner, you are potentially offering them the opportunity to learn something new.

Midwives as teachers

A recent review of the provision of antenatal education services within a large NHS trust included exploration of the views of community midwives involved in teaching classes (Bradshaw, unpublished). A questionnaire, using visual analogue scales, identified that some of the respondents felt very confident in their teaching role and found it extremely enjoyable as a result. Others painted a different picture and as the review progressed it became clear that the key issues for these midwives, involved in teaching antenatal classes, were the size of the group, training and adequate support.

Class size

Rogers (2001: 68) writes about the optimum number of people in a group. She says that the ideal size for a learning group is between 8 and 12 and that 'the larger the group, the fewer the people who will speak'. She comments that there will usually be three or four dominant individuals within a group of 19–30 people, and where there are more than 30 in the group 'little participation is possible'. An experienced teacher will split large groups into smaller groups. However, this can take up a great deal of time, particularly when teaching hands-on practical sessions such as massage or positions, where the teacher needs to provide individual attention to each client or couple. Clearly, class size is an extremely important issue. If numbers are limited appropriately, this will result in more confident teachers and an enhanced learning environment for clients (Box 5.1).

Box 5.1 Comments from midwives

'I do find the whole experience nerve-wracking because I am not used to a teaching role especially in large groups – I find big groups overwhelming.'

'It's more enjoyable to have a responsive group that gets involved – the larger the group the harder this is to achieve.'

'My lack of confidence, I feel, is not due to a lack of knowledge but more to anxiety at having to talk to a large group and lead them through a session.'

Bradshaw (unpublished)

Training and ongoing support

Community midwives are not trained teachers. Teaching adults in large groups is a skill, and like any other skill it requires training, assessment and support. Priest and Schott (2002) strongly recommend formal training for midwives, particularly in the facilitation of good interaction through group work.

A proactive, long-term approach that aims to build confidence right from the start of a midwife's career is the inclusion of a tailored module during midwifery training. For a number of years, student midwives at the University of Worcester have participated in sessions on 'How to teach adults', and 'How to prepare antenatal classes'. Their learning outcomes include the following:

- Reflect on learning and teaching theories in relation to antenatal health education.
- Plan, lead and evaluate a parenthood session within an existing programme.

Taking into account:

- adult learning theories and styles
- teaching methods
- review of recent research evidence about parenthood education
- the needs/expectations of men in relation to their role as parent.

Initial training might therefore be provided before or after registration but, whatever the case, it is important to build upon this baseline through annual updates or workshops. Ongoing support can be provided through appraisal of individual teaching sessions. The following list highlights areas for consideration during such an appraisal, where self-assessment can ideally be combined with observation by peers (Box 5.2).

Box 5.2 Sample headings for appraisal

Planning of session	Listening skills
Knowledge base	Assertiveness
Issue handling	Balancing views with those of others
Teaching men	Group/individual involvement
Use of teaching aids	Breathing techniques for labour
Body language	Massage techniques for labour
Environment	Position techniques for labour
Ease with own body	Use of environment
Use of relaxation	Aims and learning outcomes
Spoken expression	Awareness of issues
Tone of voice	Time management
Logical flow	Variety of teaching methods

NCT (2006)

NCT antenatal teachers are assessed using this method of peer observation at least once every 3 years, sometimes more often. They are all encouraged to observe other teachers annually as peer assessors, using the same method of assessment and supportive feedback. Peer observation is well established in higher education, where teachers form pairs to assess each other's practice in the classroom (Blackwell and MacLean, 1996). It is important to foster a collaborative, non-threatening, constructive and supportive approach. The aim is to enhance learning and teaching practice through an equal dialogue that fosters development of an individual's teaching skills.

Global aims

Every educator should have a global aim: this is the underpinning ethos of any individual's teaching. Educators need to spend some time reflecting upon what their 'big picture' really is and what they want their students to go away with. A clear aim should tell you what a session or course hopes to achieve. One example of a global aim is 'that the woman, her partner and their baby emerge from the birth experience feeling happy and both physically and mentally healthy'. Others might be 'that these sessions increase parents' confidence', or 'to enable parents to make informed choices' (Nolan, 1998).

Reflection

My global aim when I began to write for this chapter was 'to increase the confidence of midwives who teach antenatal classes, so that they can make the learning/teaching experience a valuable and rewarding one for both the parents who come to classes and themselves.'

Before you begin to formulate your session, think for a few moments about what your own specific wish list is for the session or course, and discuss this with those colleagues who are also involved. Ask them if they have given any thought to the bigger picture and explore the possibilities together.

Many midwives will be familiar with reflective cycle models. The following is an adaptation of Gibb's (1988) cyclical model, which can be utilised as a tool to plan a single session, or a whole course, and help you to achieve your global aims (Figure 5.1).

This cyclical approach offers a structure to work within. The first four steps emphasise the importance of planning and thorough preparation. Community midwives who are asked to teach antenatal classes need to identify that a considerable amount of time has to be set aside to prepare sessions. Negotiation is often necessary to identify some protected time in order to accomplish this. The circular process continues to highlight the role of reflection, through evaluation of the teacher's and the clients'

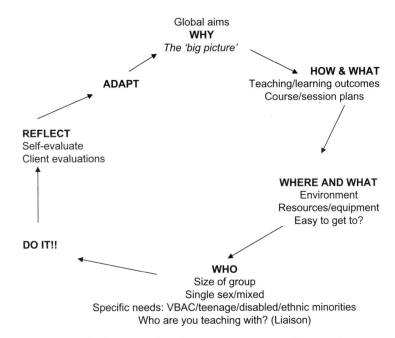

Figure 5.1 Cyclical process for planning. VBAC, vaginal birth after caesarean section.

experience of the session. Evaluation is a means of obtaining feedback that allows self-assessment of the effectiveness of our teaching. This prompts adaptations to improve teaching practice in the future. Lifelong learning is demonstrated as the cycle then begins again.

How adults learn

A sound insight into how adults learn is a pre-requisite for achieving your aims. There is a wealth of books about teaching adults, and there are numerous learning and teaching theories. Curzon (1997), in particular, suggests that teachers of 'older' students must be prepared to act as 'facilitators of learning'. Rogers (1989) states that 'all learning is best done through active involvement' and this is expanded upon by Priest and Schott (2002) who tell us that 'active involvement means the class stops being an audience and starts working as a group of people who interact with the teacher and with each other'.

A group of midwifery students were posed the question 'How do adults learn?' They compiled the following list:

Processing	Watching – listening – doing
Experience	Repetition
Interaction	By making mistakes
Conditioning	Culture and media
Reading	Reflection

The students also discussed motivation. This is one of the major differences in antenatal education, as opposed to adult education in general. There is a great deal of motivation involved. Pregnant women, and to a greater or lesser extent their partners, want to learn. They are keen to soak up information and they generally come to classes with an enormous amount of information already gleaned from the media and from their friends and family.

The really important thing to remember, when thinking about how adults learn, is that they learn best by 'doing',' so you need to use lots of different kinds of activities. These could include mini lectures, videos, group discussion (small group and large group), practising, listening to each other, games of various kinds (such as card sorting), carousels (you can use paper carousels, where you pin large sheets of paper on the wall with headings on and small groups move round to each sheet in turn writing what they know, or people carousels, where one group of people sit in a circle looking out and another group of people move around them, having 2 minutes to ask each person in the inner circle questions), role play, visitors to the group (new parents with babies), brainstorms, demonstrations, giving them tasks to do, problem-solving situations, drawing, visualisation and relaxation.

Everything needs to be kept simple. Petty (2004) urges teachers to be succinct and emphasises the need to explain and simplify. This often means missing out information that the educator may feel is important. Use key words and phrases, lists, repetition, drawings and simple diagrams.

It is also important to base your teaching on clients' prior knowledge. That means that somehow you need to find out what they already know. A straightforward approach involves brainstorming and group work before you start each topic, or use some key words and phrases and give the group/s an activity based around this.

Reflection

When I first taught antenatal classes, I always gave a lecture on pain and pain relief, giving an enormous amount of information about the effects of drugs during labour. Over time, I have moved toward giving groups the information on handouts, and letting them present the pros and cons of each. Now I often just stick flip chart paper around the room with headings such as 'Water', 'Massage', 'Gas and air', 'Pethidine/Meptid', etc.

I split the class into small groups, give them some coloured pens, and then I leave them to it. After 20 minutes I usually find that I hardly need to say anything; I can just draw out the relevant links or gently correct any incorrect information.

Most clients who come to antenatal classes already know a huge amount about pregnancy, birth and parenting. They have probably seen a number of births on Sky TV. They have amassed knowledge from their friends and family, soaked up the predominant culture of childbirth within their family and community, and they have already made many decisions. This vast amount of information and prior knowledge can be explored and fine tuned by presenting research-based information in understandable terms. Aim to provide clear, straightforward answers to questions. Discussion with others in the group, and practical work on whatever topic you are covering, encourages the ongoing process of active learning that will feed into informed decision-making.

Planning a session

Putting a session together starts with compiling the learning outcomes and then planning how to teach the session in some detail. Whether you are responsible for a whole course of classes, or just one session, you will need to sit down and work out exactly what you are going to teach, how you are going to teach it and what your learning outcomes will be. It is essential that midwives who teach antenatal classes have clear learning outcomes because learning outcomes are measurable through evaluation. Evaluation offers the potential to link the impact of antenatal classes to birth outcomes and hopefully in the future we will be able to demonstrate that effective antenatal education can make a difference.

Learning outcomes

The formulation of learning outcomes begins with focusing on the key issues. If the first stage of labour is used as an example, the key issues could include three coping techniques for labour: staying upright, relaxing and being mobile. These topics have been used as a basis to state what the teacher is aiming for by the end of the session (Box 5.3).

Box 5.3 Learning outcomes example

By the end of this class clients will:

- **know** what the benefits of upright positions in labour are and how this affects the physiology of labour
- be able to **demonstrate** a range of upright positions
- be able to **describe** the effects and **enumerate** the benefits of being relaxed on the hormones that drive labour
- be able to **identify** different practical relaxation techniques
- **interpret** how mobility in labour affects the pelvis and, in turn, facilitates the baby's passage through it.

Note that the above learning outcomes incorporate a number of active verbs. These relate to the acquisition of knowledge, the understanding of that knowledge and how it can be applied. Learning outcomes are not always easy to compile, but they are very worthwhile. They focus the mind, offer structure and add a professional dimension to your teaching.

Always keep in mind that antenatal education must be driven by the needs of the clients and what they want to learn. Priest and Schott (2002) warn that learning outcomes can easily be biased to meet the objectives of the teacher, resulting in failure to meet parents' needs. Nolan (1998) echoes this in stating that 'the only way to select the most appropriate topics from the multiplicity of topics that could be covered during an antenatal course is to ask the group members what they most want to learn about'.

A great fear is that, if you ask women and their birth partners, they might want something very different to what you have planned for them. If your sessions have specific learning outcomes and you have put together a balanced and interesting session you will find that, for the most part, what clients ask for will already be included. It also helps if you give your sessions a meaningful title. If a session is called 'Coping skills for labour' then it is obvious that it is not going to cover any baby care and that it is going to be a relatively practical session. In fact, it could be renamed 'Practical skills for labour' or 'Powers and passage – practically perfect birthing skills' and still convey a clear meaning in relation to the proposed content. Think not only about how the sessions are presented, but how they are titled. If you are leading a whole course then rather than 'The antenatal classes', why not have different titles for each session. Clients will then have a good idea about what is going to be presented before they arrive and it is highly likely that the learning outcomes for the session will fit in with their expectations.

Learning and teaching styles

Rogers (1989) reminds us that all learning is best done through active involvement and it must be remembered that individuals have different preferred learning styles. Learning styles have been categorised since the 1970s. There are numerous models to choose from, one being reported by Grinder (1993), who describes four types of learner: visual, auditory, kinaesthetic and tactile. It is quite possible for individuals to hold strong preferences for more than one of these modalities. In principle, when learning styles are identified, educators can take these into consideration and tailor their teaching to facilitate effective learning. When teaching groups, it is clearly impractical to identify the preferred learning style for every single individual. However, if you use as many different ways of teaching as you can, not only will your sessions be more interesting, but you will be teaching far more effectively by addressing a good mix of learning styles.

When I put my sessions together, I have to remember that I enjoy telling a story, acting it out and being the centre of attention. As a result, I have to make sure that I consciously plan to use a wide range of teaching styles and only use my actress role when it is the right moment to do so. Think about what your preferred style is – and think about how you can vary it.

Sometimes it helps to draw a spidergram or a flow chart, or just simply write down what you want to do in the order you want to do it. Then, using a different coloured pen, write against each item the amount of time that you want to spend on this topic or activity. Using another different coloured pen, write against each item one of the following words:

practical	discussion	lecture	group work
ice breaker	relaxation	single-sex discussion	men's needs
video	role play	game	carousel
demonstration			

This list is not exhaustive! But remember that most people learn best by *doing*.

This will help you to define your preferred teaching style and then vary it. Many of us find safety in lecturing, where we stand or sit in a position of authority in a classroom-style setting. One good example, demonstrating how easy it is to revert to the safety of lecturing, is the postnatal 'goody bag'. How many teachers pass the bag (or bucket) around and let class members take items out and talk about what they think they are and what they are used for? And how many fall into the trap of standing at the front of the group, taking out each item and giving a mini-lecture on each one? It is obvious which of these strategies is the more active and enjoyable approach for participants. The former facilitates visual, auditory and tactile learning styles. Increasing involvement means that learning will be more effective.

Focusing down and managing time

Perhaps the biggest mistake when planning a session or a course is under-estimating the amount of time needed for a topic. A session on the first stage of labour is a good example. Is this an easy topic to teach in an hour or two? It might seem possible, until you begin to list or build a spidergram of what needs to be included:

- physiology – what is happening?
- things to watch out for – 'what to do if. . . .'
- start of labour – how do I know I'm in labour?

- when to go into hospital (hospital birth)
- when to call the midwife (home birth)
- what to take with me
- what to do while I am at home in early labour
- pain – what is normal; what to expect
- pain control/relief: self help or drugs?
- practical coping skills: positions; massage; movement; breathing
- partner's needs?
- induction
- acceleration

. . . and lots more!

This is the moment when panic can set in! How can you possibly cover all of this information within 2 hours? The answer is simple: you can't.

When I first began teaching for the NCT many years ago, I had the luxury of 8 weeks of 2-hour sessions. Now I teach labour days, and sometimes half days. When I recently led workshops for a local community midwifery team, I taught 'Coping skills for labour' in one afternoon. When you have only a small amount of time available, you have to focus down to what women and their partners really need to know.

So, if your friend is due to have her baby any day now and she is off to Scotland on a train, what three things does she need to know about labour? What three things can you tell her that she can remember as she rushes to get onto the train? Staying upright, relaxing and keeping mobile all spring to mind. We will all think of three different things, but in the main we will be thinking along the same lines. Treat every topic that you are going to teach in this same way – keep it simple, keep it focused – think about what your clients actually need to know to get somewhere near your global aims.

Putting it together – step by step example

Let's take the example of a 2-hour session for women and their partners where the topic is the first stage of labour.

Step 1

Take a few minutes to either write out your global aim for the session or reconnect with this if you have one already. Ask yourself 'What is my deepest wish/desire for these couples?' One example might be something along the lines of 'They will understand enough about the physiology of labour to be able to effectively utilise positions, movement and non-pharmacological coping techniques and have straightforward vaginal births – and if they experience a complicated, surgical birth they will understand the reasons why and be strengthened by the knowledge that they did everything they could to make as much space as possible for the baby.'

Step 2
Put together a few learning outcomes. You can come back to them and refine them when you have planned the whole session. Ask yourself the question 'What do I want the class to be able to do/know by the end of the session – and can this be measured?' Remember to use active verbs when formulating the learning outcomes to ensure that they are measurable through evaluation.

Step 3
Focus down to identify the key points that clients need to know about the first stage of labour. Take each topic and think about how you are going to teach/facilitate/demonstrate this. Use a mix of teaching methods. If you find it helps, colour code each topic using a different colour for lecture, brainstorm, video, etc. If there's too much pink, for example, and you have used pink for lecturing, then you have too much lecturing in your session. For the first stage of labour, I might build the session around using the following four statements: keep upright; keep forward; keep mobile; keep smiling.

This would be the bare minimum for a really short session. The beauty of focusing right down like this is that you can then expand it all out again as much or as little as you need – you have control.

Keep upright: Demonstrate why this is beneficial in labour. Show the group a pelvis and a doll – let them hold them and pass them around. What happens to the pelvis and the position of the baby when you sit down or lie down? Hold the pelvis in front of you to demonstrate lying on your back, push a coconut through to represent the baby's head – you're pushing up a 1 in 5 gradient against gravity. You're squashing your tailbone. It's going to hurt and take a long time. Hold the pelvis upright, and the coconut drops out! This is very effective and visual. There are lots of other ways of doing this – you can use a grapefruit instead of a coconut or you could use a tumble drier hose. The hose is a brilliant prop that lends itself to demonstrate how the vaginal walls unfold during the second stage of labour.

Explain that it's the weight of the baby's head on the cervix (that's the bit like a tightly closed polo-neck jumper that keeps the baby sealed inside – it has to open for the baby to move down into the vagina) that makes the brain produce lots of petrol (oxytocin) to fire the uterus up and keep good, effective contractions going. You can use analogies such as describing being upright as being the same as putting your foot on the accelerator in the car (Jowitt, 1993).

Keep forward: Explain why. Tell the group that the uterus lifts upward and forwards when it contracts. Sit back in your chair or lie on the floor and demonstrate a forward motion with your hands. Ask the group 'Is this harder work in these positions?' Tell them yes – it is going to hurt more. Stand up, lean forward against the wall and let them see how much easier the work is for the uterus in this position. Let parents learn that working with their bodies makes labour more efficient, and reduces pain. You might then link this to the fear–tension–pain cycle (see Nolan, 1998).

Keep mobile: Why? Because labouring women are often restless and need to move around; babies need to be 'shifted on down' into the pelvis. If women are mobile they can lunge, they can circle their hips and they can go up and down stairs sideways. They can do whatever they like! At this point I often do a belly-dancing session. This is great fun, acts as an icebreaker and demonstrates mobility as a coping technique. Pain is a message from the baby to *do* something. When a young relative of mine had her first baby, she didn't go to any classes and then laboured at home, on her own, until she got to 8 cm. I asked her what she did to cope, and she said 'I just leant again the wall and the sofa and circled my hips – it seemed the right thing to do'.

Keep smiling: Why? Well, women need to feel at ease with their environment to labour naturally. Explain the intricate hormonal dance between a woman and her baby – ask the group what happens when you feel anxious and uncomfortable. What hormone do you produce? Hopefully, someone will shout out the answer 'adrenalin' and you can ask them what they think the effect of adrenalin in first stage of labour might be. You have now laid the groundwork to link to the topic of relaxation techniques.

Step 4

Continue with all that you want to include in your session, breaking it into small topics and then focusing each topic down into three or four important key points. Make sure that you build in time at the beginning of the session for introductions and icebreakers, and prioritise to allow time for a break halfway through. You will also need time at the end for evaluations, questions and clearing up.

Step 5

Now transfer everything to a format that you can glance at or follow whilst you are teaching. You might just list the main topics and key words against them; you might draw bubbles with arrows linking them; you may have a computer programme that you can use. You may feel you need to write notes on everything you want to say or do. Some teachers use a card system. There is no right or wrong way to do this – you need to find the most effective format for you.

Tips for teachers

Teaching is a daunting task for many community midwives but once you gain some experience the unthinkable often happens as the 'doing it' bit starts to feel exciting and enjoyable. If you have a basic structure to your session then you can enjoy the process. Try to keep relaxed, keep it simple, include plenty of group activities and throw difficult questions back to the group. For those midwives who find teaching difficult, or who are just plain terrified, key messages are summarised in Box 5.4.

Box 5.4 Tips for the terrified

- Keep your sessions simple and focused.
- Above all, remember what you are trying to achieve. What is your global aim? Feel passionate about it and let your beliefs colour how you teach and speak.
- Persuade your team leader to let you teach smaller groups. This can be achieved by doing fewer, more focused sessions, or by adopting case load classes. If you have to teach large groups, make sure you split them into small groups and give them lots of group work to do.
- Class members are likely to be nervous as well – they do not know what to expect or what they are letting themselves in for. Men, in particular, are usually uncomfortable at the first class.
- Have your teaching session set out on paper (or on cards) beside you. Use large type so that you can see it clearly.
- Give them plenty to do; the more you give the class to do the less you have to be the centre of attention. Use lots of handouts and lots of practical sessions. During a massage session you can walk around and do lots of on-the-spot teaching to individual couples/clients.
- Have plenty of back-up teaching tricks up your sleeve as a fall-back plan for moments of panic.
- Throw questions, particularly awkward ones, back to the group.
- Don't be afraid to say you don't know the answer to something, but promise to find out and remember to carry that promise out.
- Practise over and over again any activity that you need to demonstrate, so that you feel more at ease, e.g. demonstrating positions.
- Consider the language that you are going to use; don't use technical jargon. Use ordinary terms that people can identify with and that you feel comfortable using.
- Watch your body language – you may be saying one thing but your body language may be saying something different.

Remember that men often feel very uncomfortable in the class because they are anxious and unsure of what to expect. Consciously aim your teaching toward the men and birth supporters in the group because they are the people who can help the woman most. Show them how to massage, let them hold the pelvis and ask them to think about what happens to the baby if the woman lies down, stands up or leans forward. Allow men time together as a single sex group with some fun activities. My favourite is 'naming the parts of a woman's body'. Use small cards with Velcro backings for them to stick onto a large diagram. You can also try the 'seeing how much you can get into a pair of tights' activity (Box 5.5). Give them a pair of tights and ask them to fill them with rice, water, sugar and flour from the following list, after having tied knots in each leg of the tights just under the crotch area.

Box 5.5 Shopping list for 'seeing how much you can get into a pair of tights'

- 3 litre plastic bottle of cooking oil (fat deposits during pregnancy)
- 4 kg bag of rice (a fairly large baby)
- 1 litre of water in a tightly sealed freezer bag (amniotic fluid)
- 500 g bag of sugar (placenta)
- 1 kg bag of flour (uterus)
- 500 g bag of pasta (breasts)
- 2 litre bottle of water (extra fluid in blood and tissues)

This is a fun exercise that also helps partners to understand just what happens to a woman's physiology during pregnancy. It can be linked to topics in other sessions such as blood loss during the third stage of labour. It is also very useful for introducing the topic of pelvic floor exercises for both men and women.

Groups will need to choose a spokesperson to feedback from activities. This feedback will help you to assess how well you explained the task and whether the activity was relevant and appropriate. Group work is invariably successful if you have organised your materials and resources well and kept it simple.

The where, what and who?

For most community midwives, the organisational and logistical aspects of teaching classes are not under their control, but it is important to ask the following key questions:

- Where are you teaching?
- What resources are available?
- Who are you teaching?

The environment in which you teach is as important for you as it is for your clients. People will only learn if they are comfortable in their surroundings. How can you do small group work if you teach in an antenatal clinic with fixed seating? How can you teach effectively and professionally if your dolls are battered and tatty, and your pelvis is falling apart? How can you show videos or DVDs if you only have a tiny TV set that hardly anyone in the room can see? Realistically, most of us have to work with what we have, but try to look around where you teach with a critical eye to see if you could make some changes in the environment. Remember that smells can affect individuals on a subconscious level, particularly if you are teaching in a hospital-based environment. The simple measure of changing the smell of a room can make an enormous difference to first impressions and how clients feel. Consider taking some bowls of pot pourri or an aromatherapy air freshener with you. If you are able to do so safely, you might burn a scented candle but make sure that the smells are not too strong or intrusive. Choose scents such as lemon and peppermint, which keep people's minds active. A few fresh flowers in a vase and some bowls of chocolates placed around the room are touches that demonstrate to clients that they are valued and that you want them to feel comfortable. Add some gentle background music – 'womb sound' type music is fun and will often start discussions about babies and what they can hear and do whilst in the womb.

If the room in which you teach is truly dreadful then put pressure on your team leader to try and find somewhere more suitable or look for an alternative yourself. The new children's centres are increasingly being utilised as very appropriate local venues. Maslow's (1954) hierarchy of needs tells us about differing levels or layers of need that have to be met for adults to learn effectively. On a practical level this means a number of things. Pregnant women will definitely need comfortable seating and a reasonable temperature in the room. They need access to drinks and to food (chocolates, biscuits, dried fruit and fresh fruit are all good – you can ask them to bring their own). These are the very basics that need to be provided. The next layer is safety and security. Clients need to have a good idea of the structure of the session and when breaks are scheduled. They also need to know where the toilets are and that they can leave the group for a comfort break at any time without having to advertise the fact by putting their hand up to ask for permission. They need to know what to bring with them to the session. If you have asked the group to bring pillows, for example, always bring a couple of spare ones yourself. You can let forgetful clients use these and the feelings of embarrassment and panic will then be avoided when they realise they have forgotten to bring their own pillows with them. Confidentiality within the group should be negotiated and some teachers ask the group to put together their own ground rules. All that you do to make the environment right for teaching is very similar to what we should be doing to make the birth environment relaxing and homely. Your feelings and beliefs about a woman's needs in labour are often reflected in the way you teach.

Before you teach, you need some basic information about the nature of the client group. You cannot plan your session without knowing exactly who you are going to be teaching. For instance, if you have a teenage group, then you need to make certain that your sessions are geared toward that group's specific needs. Remember above all that clients come to classes with their own expectations and agendas, and that most have their own internal, often subconscious, dream of how they want their birth experience to be. It is unrealistic to think that you will meet every woman's needs in one particular session. You are not going to make a big difference for everybody who comes to your class and it is important to remember this point, because after you have taught each session and reviewed the evaluation forms it will help you to maintain a logical perspective.

Reflection and evaluation

Make sure that evaluations are completed by both the women and their birth partners at the end of the session. If you ask for them to be returned later, you are unlikely to get all of them back. Try to print evaluation forms on coloured paper rather than white. Lemon or pink forms are supposedly more likely to be completed. Keep it short and simple, and only ask for what you want to know, for example:

- Did you enjoy the class?
- What have you learnt?
- Would you change anything – add something, or take something away?
- Would you recommend the class to someone else?

The format of your evaluation forms will evolve as you identify the issues pertinent to your situation. If you want more detailed feedback about the effectiveness of your teaching, you might devise a Likert-type scale. More recently I have given out an evaluation form that has half-completed statements, and this seems to be working very well because the responses are much more meaningful:

I feel ....
Today I found out that ....

Today I felt ....
I feel really good about ....
My next step is ....
I want to say that ....
Today this group has given me ....
My positive intention is ....

Reading evaluations can occasionally be soul-destroying. One way to cope with negative feedback – 'the biscuits were rubbish!' – is to count up the total number of responses and work out how many agreed that the biscuits were rubbish. Then turn these responses into a percentage. Often you find that only 2% of the responses agreed with this statement, so it is irrelevant. If you find that 98% of the responses say the biscuits were rubbish, then clearly you need to change the biscuits, bearing in mind that the next group may not like the new ones!

Self-evaluation and reflection is vitally important and part of the cycle that will facilitate your development as a teacher. Sometimes it has to be done on the spot. You can tell if something isn't going well and you might need to change and adapt on your feet as you are teaching. Alternatively, you need to sit back after the class to think about how you can approach a particular exercise the next time. Constantly change and adapt to continue your own learning, but try new activities on at least two groups before you make major changes. Sometimes it isn't you: it just hasn't worked for that particular group.

Summary

You might already be aware of a process called 'deep learning'. This occurs when someone's whole internalised concept of something is gradually changed over a period of time because of what they have absorbed subconsciously from a teacher or mentor. It goes beyond the mere acquisition of factual knowledge and it frequently results in a change in behaviour. This is where your global aims and passion illuminate your individual 'big picture'. Identify your passions before you begin to teach, let them colour everything you say and do and your knowledge and enthusiasm will be infectious.

My passions can be summed up as internalised beliefs that the majority of women *can* give birth vaginally. They can learn active birth techniques that maximise the likelihood of this normal outcome. These passions are what inspire me to teach and they remain unchanged because I believe in them. I will have achieved my global aim for this chapter if readers are encouraged to identify their own passions and then subsequently translate them into words and action.

Finally, how do you end a session/class? Simply say:

'Thank you for being here: it's time to go home now'.

⚷ Key points

- Expectant parents are highly motivated to learn.
- Channelling your passion about birth illuminates learning and teaching.
- Planning your teaching increases confidence and effectiveness.
- Adults learn best in a safe and comfortable environment.
- Adults learn best when they are actively involved – remember the golden rules: get them *talking*, get them *thinking*, get them *doing*.

References

Blackwell, R. and MacLean, M. (1996) Peer observation of teaching and staff development. *Higher Education Quarterly*, **50** (2), 156–171.

Curzon, L.B. (1997) *Teaching in Further Education: An Outline of Principles and Practice*, 5th edn. Cassell, London.

Gibbs, G. (1988) *Learning by Doing: A Guide to Teaching and Learning Methods.* Oxford Polytechnic, Oxford Further Education Unit.

Ginnis, P. (2004) *Teacher's Toolkit: Raise Classroom Achievement with Strategies for Every Learner*. Crown House, Carmarthen.

Grinder, M. (1993) *ENVOY: Your Personal Guide to Classroom Management*. Michael *Grinder* and Associates, Washington.

Jowitt, M. (1993) *Childbirth Unmasked*. Peter Wooller, Craven Arms.

Maslow, A.H. (1954) *Motivation and Personality*. Harper and Row, New York.

NCT (2006) *Assessment Grid*. National Childbirth Trust, London.

Nolan, M. (1998) *Antenatal Education: A Dynamic Approach*. Balliere Tindall, London.

Petty, G. (2004) *Teaching Today*, 3rd edn. Nelson Thornes, Cheltenham.

Priest, J. and Schott, J. (2002) *Leading Antenatal Classes: A Practical Guide*, 2nd edn. Books for Midwives, Oxford.

Rogers, J. (1989) *Adults Learning*, 3rd edn. Open University Press, Milton Keynes.

Rogers, J. (2001) *Adults Learning*, 4th edn. Open University Press, Milton Keynes.

Babies

Newborn screening revisited: what midwives need to know

Nadia Permalloo and Jean Chapple

For three decades, midwifery practice has included the screening of newborn babies as an integral part of care, so why are we devoting a whole chapter to it? Changes in both midwifery practice and screening programmes make an update timely, for example the current climate in which midwives practise makes it unacceptable to perform a test without obtaining informed consent, while the publication of new and revised national standards and implementation of newer programmes such as screening for cystic fibrosis (CF) or sickle cell disorders (SCD) mean that midwives need to know more detail about screening programmes to detect more diseases. Midwives need to ensure they have the knowledge, skills and attitude to deliver midwifery care fit for the 21st century.

This chapter provides community midwives with knowledge about the basic principles of screening, examines the conditions currently offered in newborn screening programmes and the rationale and national standards underpinning those programmes. It explores the midwife's role in reducing risk in an area where errors can easily occur because of the various components, systems and professionals involved.

Principles of screening

When midwives hear the term 'screening', they may think of complex technical tests but screening is embedded in basic midwifery practice. At every encounter with the mother and baby, a midwife screens by careful observation, looking for signs of 'normality' and/or any deviation so that they can give or refer for appropriate care. Whenever a midwife palpates a woman's abdomen, she is screening for intrauterine growth restriction. Every time she takes a woman's blood pressure or tests her urine, she is screening for pre-eclampsia. Every time a midwife 'checks the baby over' in the newborn period, she is screening for conditions such as jaundice.

There are other elements of care that midwives deliver that they may be tempted to classify as screening. For example, when a midwife is in the woman's home skilfully observing the dynamics of the family relationships, she may also notice signs of domestic abuse, child protection issues and everyday safety concerns. This is not screening because it is not performed in any systematic way. Mezey and Bewley (1997) describe this approach as 'case finding' and there may not be any clear pathways for successful intervention to improve the situation. Case finding involves clinicians looking for illness or its predictors whenever a patient presents to them for another reason.

The National Screening Committee (NSC) (DH, 2000) defines screening as 'a public health service in which members of a defined population, who do not necessarily perceive they are at risk of, or are already affected by, a disease or its complications, are asked a question or offered a test to identify those individuals who are more likely to be helped than harmed by further tests or treatment to reduce the risk of disease or its complications'.

The NSC's mission statement is to 'use research evidence to identify programmes that do more good than harm at a reasonable cost' (NSC, 2006a), reminding us that screening has the potential to damage health as well as improve it. Trying to get the right balance between good and harm is challenging, as no two families will use the same decision-making process. Abramsky (2003) describes prenatal screening as a double-edged sword that can do good and harm, often at the same time to the same person. Later in the chapter we will discuss further practical steps the midwife can take to ensure that parents are fully informed.

In addition to everyday midwifery tasks, there are other more formal tests that are offered to parents (e.g. newborn hearing screening), but there is an important distinction between screening tests and screening programmes. It can be very harmful to implement a screening test without the infrastructure needed to support your action. For example:

- Would there be any value in screening for congenital hypothyroidism (CHT) if thyroxine was not available to treat those babies with the condition?
- What are the consequences of screening for SCD without the parents realising that it is an inherited disease?
- What would happen if a new member of staff did not offer screening for CF as it was not offered at her previous place of employment and she had not been trained to undertake the procedure?

If any components of a screening programme are not provided, harm can ensue. We need to implement screening programmes, not just screening tests. The components that are essential for a good screening programme are:

- There should be an education programme for all professionals, including support staff (such as interpreters) involved in delivering the programme. This includes information and an awareness programme for the audience you are going to offer screening to – in this case women, parents and their families.
- There should be a robust system for collecting the samples/conducting tests and ensuring they reach their destination, for example a laboratory where they will be analysed.
- There should be a quality assurance system to ensure that tests are carried out to a defined standard and are reproducible, i.e. to ensure that a laboratory produces the same result on the same sample as another laboratory elsewhere in the country and deals with samples in a timely fashion.
- There should be a system for ensuring that women/parents receive the results, including negative (normal) results. The policy of 'no news is good news' does not fulfil the criteria of a screening programme and, more importantly, the needs of parents.
- For positive (abnormal) results there needs to be a clear pathway, including information and counselling, the option to have further confirmatory or diagnostic tests, treatment and additional support as appropriate.
- There should be a system for capturing all stages of the pathway and the decisions taken: good information systems are vital. The information system not only allows you to record information but should have the functionality for you to retrieve data as required to enable adequate monitoring of the screening programme.

A good screening test is part of a good screening programme. It should be both sensitive (able to pick up most cases of the disorder) and specific (able to correctly rule out those people without the disorder). If a screening test is not sensitive, many cases will be missed. If it is not specific, then there will be many 'false positive/abnormal' results and people without the disease will have been worried and investigated unnecessarily. Fortunately, all tests used in the newborn period are both relatively sensitive and specific.

It is very important to understand that screening does not give parents a definitive answer and requires further test(s) in order to confirm the diagnosis. If you are asked to visit to repeat a blood spot sample, you should ensure that you know the reasons why this repeat has been requested. It may be that the initial sample was inadequate but it may very well be that it is to confirm the initial finding. If you receive a request for a repeat sample you need to take action urgently and ensure you know why the repeat has been requested in order to inform the parents appropriately.

The National Screening Committee

The UK NSC was established in 1996 and advises Ministers, the devolved National Assemblies and the Scottish Parliament on related issues. These include the case for implementing new population screening pro-grammes and the appraisal of screening technologies of proven effective-ness but which require controlled and well-managed introduction.

The committee also reviews the case for continuing, modifying or withdrawing existing population screening programmes, in particular programmes inadequately evaluated or of doubtful effectiveness, quality or value.

The NSC performs its functions by assessing screening programmes against a set of internationally recognised criteria (Wilson and Jungner, 1968; Cochrane and Holland, 1971; Cuckle and Wald, 1984). Situations where there are clear benefits for screening are:

- a well-defined disease with clear diagnostic criteria
- a known natural history – we know what will happen to an indi-vidual with the disease
- important health problems for the individual and for the commu-nity, as it is either severe, common or both
- known incidence and prevalence in the community
- the condition is preventable by acceptable methods.

The NSC currently oversees over 100 screening programmes where assessment against the above criteria has resulted in a screening policy decision. There is also an ongoing plan to review all these policies in light of new evidence that may arise. The Screening Specialist Library is an online source of the latest information on any possible screening programme in the UK (NSC, 2006b).

For each of the screening programmes, the NSC sets national stan-dards that local programmes are required to achieve. This ensures that local programmes are in line with the best available evidence, avoids a postcode lottery of screening and ensures equal access across the country so that wherever a woman books for care or has her baby she is offered the same package of care and the quality of care is comparable.

The rationale for newborn screening

Screening newborn infants is extremely important as it significantly reduces associated morbidity and mortality by ensuring that treatment and appropriate interventions are put in place in a timely manner. This not only has implications for the individual child but also has a wider impact on the public health agenda. Currently, there is wide discussion about the role of the midwife in public health but many midwives are not clear about what this means or how it may influence their future role and function.

The government has set a target as part of its inequalities agenda, 'To reduce inequalities in health outcomes by 10% by 2010 as measured by infant mortality and life expectancy at birth' (DH, 2003). Reidpath and Allotey (2003) describe infant mortality as a sensitive measure of the overall health of a population. It reflects the apparent association between the causes of infant mortality and other factors that are likely to influence the health status of whole populations, such as their economic development, general living conditions, social well-being, rates of illness and the quality of the environment.

If we unpick the two statements above it will become apparent that the midwife has a central role and function to play in achieving the government's target and improving infant health for every baby. This role is not limited to the midwife's role in antenatal and newborn screening, but the government does indicate key interventions that will achieve the desired outcome and the majority are dependent on the full participation of midwives. These include pre-conceptual care, including early folic acid supplementation, access to antenatal care, smoking cessation, prevention of sudden infant death, teenage pregnancies and breastfeeding. All of these areas of midwifery practice predominantly involve midwives who are working in the community. They need to take up the challenge of their role in the wider public health agenda by reviewing working patterns, breaking down barriers caused by professional demarcations and working as a cohesive team to deliver appropriate packages of care to women, parents and their babies.

The newborn screening programmes currently implemented in the UK are:

- newborn blood spot including:
  - phenylketonuria (PKU)
  - congenital hypothyroidism (CHT)
  - sickle cell disorders (SCD)
  - medium chain acyl-coA dehydrogenase deficiency (MCADD)
  - cystic fibrosis (CF)
- newborn hearing screening
- newborn and 6–8 week infant physical examination.

Newborn blood spot screening

Newborn blood spot screening is the oldest and arguably the most successful screening programme in the UK. Every parent in the UK is offered the chance to find out if their child has been born with a disease which, if left untreated, would permanently affect their child's health. The success of the programme means that children with PKU now remain well enough to form partnerships and have their own families. Before screening was introduced, affected children formed a sizable proportion of the populations of large residential institutions for people with severe learning disabilities.

Babies cannot be tested until they are physiologically separate from their mother and producing their own proteins and hormones. This occurs by the fifth day of life (the date of birth is counted as day 0). As treatment for both PKU and CHT must be started as quickly as possible to prevent permanent brain damage, blood spots (which are used for screening all conditions) are taken onto specially treated cards between day 5 and day 8 to allow the programme to identify affected babies by day 19 and for treatment to be initiated by day 21.

Bloodspot cards are analysed by tandem mass spectrometry – potentially this laboratory development could pick up over 200 inherited metabolic disorders but most are extremely rare and incurable and do not therefore meet the criteria for a disease screening programme.

Phenylketonuria

Our bodies need to breakdown phenylalanine, an amino acid found in proteins to produce tyrosine which is essential for brain development. For this conversion to be achieved the enzyme phenylalanine hydroxylase is required. Babies with PKU are unable to metabolise phenylalanine due to a lack of phenylalanine hydroxylase. The production of phenylalanine hydroxylase is controlled by a gene on chromosome 12. PKU is an autosomal recessive genetic condition and therefore both parents who carry the unusual gene will have a one in four chance of having an affected child in each pregnancy. Adults are not screened for PKU carrier status so in most cases parents will only discover they have an unusual gene when their child is diagnosed with the condition. Parents who already have an affected child and therefore know their carrier status can choose to have prenatal diagnosis in subsequent pregnancies.

PKU was first described in 1934 by a Norwegian doctor called Folling when a mother of two children with learning disabilities expressed concern that her children had a peculiar smell. Dr Folling found phenylketones in the urine of the two children, hence the name phenylketonuria. The National Newborn Screening Programme for PKU was introduced in 1969 and is known as the Guthrie test after Robert Guthrie, microbiologist and paediatrician at the State University of New York, Buffalo, who developed a blood test for PKU to replace the previous practice of testing wet nappies. The term 'Guthrie test' is no longer accurate for describing blood spot screening as it only relates to PKU and the blood spot screening programme now includes four other conditions (Box 6.1).

Box 6.1 Key messages: phenylketonuria

- PKU is an autosomal recessive genetic condition that affects 1 in 10000 babies in the UK.
- Babies with this condition are unable to metabolise phenylalanine (an amino acid found in proteins).
- Untreated babies develop serious, permanent learning difficulties.
- Screen-positive babies are seen by a specialist and a low protein diet should be started by 21 days of age: treatment is very effective.
- Ongoing treatment, with a strictly controlled diet, prevents disability.

Further information

National Society for PKU www.nspku.org.

Screening brief: Phenylketonuria. *Journal of Medical Screening* **6**, 113, 1999.

Congenital hypothyroidism

CHT is a disorder affecting the thyroid gland, and the National Newborn Screening Programme for CHT was introduced in 1981. The thyroid gland produces a chemical called thyroxine, which is essential for normal growth and development. Hypothyroidism occurs if the thyroid gland does not produce enough thyroxine. CHT is present at birth and prevents normal brain development. Babies with a normal thyroid at birth may develop hypothyroidism much later in life but the effects of this are much less pronounced once the brain has already fully developed.

There are several reasons why the thyroid gland may not produce enough thyroxine at birth. The gland may be completely absent or partly developed or there may be an error at some point in the hormone production pathway (Box 6.2).

Box 6.2 Key messages: congenital hypothyroidism

- CHT affects 1 in 4000 babies in the UK.
- Babies with this condition produce insufficient thyroxine.
- Untreated babies develop permanent physical and mental disability.
- Screen-positive babies are seen by a specialist and treatment with thyroxine should be started by 21 days of age.
- Treatment is effective in preventing severe learning disability.

Further information

Great Ormond Street Hospital for Children NHS Trust (GOSH) and UCL Institute of Child Health (ICH) http://www.gosh.nhs.uk/factsheets/families/F040274/index.html.

Screening brief: Screening for congenital hypothyroidism. *Journal of Medical Screening* **7**, 212, 2000.

Sickle cell disorders

SCDs include sickle cell anaemia and SC disease, SD^{Punjab}, $SB^{thalassaemia}$ and haemoglobin SO^{Arab}. All newborn infants in England are now screened for SCDs as part of the newborn blood spot screening programme. This programme was phased in from 2003 and achieved complete coverage across England in 2006. Screening allows early detection and appropriate interventions to prevent significant mortality in these children. Children with SCDs may develop sudden severe overwhelming infections. Early diagnosis allows prophylactic treatment with penicillin and pneumococcal vaccines, and parent training to identify complications.

SCDs are autosomal recessive genetic conditions, so both parents who carry the unusual gene will have a one in four chance of having an affected child in each pregnancy. All pregnant women in areas with a high prevalence of SCDs (more than 1.5 affected fetuses per 10 000 pregnancies) and in low prevalence areas those identified by a 'family origin questionnaire' as being at risk are offered antenatal screening for SCDs and thalassaemia in the UK (NHS Sickle Cell and Thalassaemia Screening Programme, 2003). If the woman is found to be a carrier for an SCD (sometimes known as sickle cell trait), the father of her baby is offered screening. If he is also a carrier, then the couple can be offered an antenatal diagnostic test. Links between the antenatal and newborn screening programmes are helpful in monitoring both programmes and familiarising parents with their carrier status but may, very rarely, disclose non-paternity (Box 6.3).

Box 6.3 Key messages: sickle cell disorders

- Sickle cell disorders affect 1 in 2500 babies in the UK.
- Affected babies are treated with penicillin and pneumococcal (Prevenar) vaccine before 3 months of age.
- Untreated babies are at high risk of death or complications from treatable infections or severe acute anaemia in the first few years of life.
- Parents of affected children need to be fully informed and involved in the management of their child's condition.
- The newborn screening programme tests for SCDs only – unlike the antenatal programme, it does not screen for thalassaemia.
- The newborn screening programme for SCDs is designed to pick up unaffected babies who are carriers of SCDs. This information will be useful to these babies when they grow up and have their own children.

Further information
Sickle Cell Society www.sicklecellsociety.org.

Medium chain acyl CoA dehydrogenase deficiency

MCADD was first described in 1982. MCADD is another autosomal recessive inherited condition and the gene for MCADD is located on chromosome 1. Similar to PKU in that it is caused by the lack of an enzyme, in this instance the enzyme is required for metabolising fat into energy. Complications present when children with MCADD have long fasting periods or an infection and have to call on their fat reserves to produce energy. They can break these down but do so inefficiently due to the lack of medium chain acyl CoA dehydrogenase. Children can quickly become hypoglycaemic. In addition, the 'banked up' medium chain fats form toxic substances, which can lead to serious life-threatening symptoms and death. Screening for MCADD currently occurs as a pilot project across 50% of England but will shortly be introduced across the UK (Box 6.4).

Box 6.4 Key messages: medium chain acyl CoA dehydrogenase deficiency

- MCADD is an autosomal recessive genetic condition that affects 1:10000–20000 babies in the UK. Mean age at presentation is 14 months.
- MCADD affects breakdown of fat and blocks energy production. This can result in drowsiness, lethargy, vomiting and seizures, and in some cases coma and death.
- 20–25% mortality: 30% of survivors will have central nervous system sequelae.
- Symptoms can occur quickly in infants who are not feeding well or are unwell with an intercurrent infection, such as diarrhoea and vomiting.
- Treatment is by prevention of metabolic crisis: avoid fasting and employ close monitoring to determine safe periods between meals.
- Implement emergency regime if unwell. This involves administration of a glucose polymer ('Maxijul') and intravenous dextrose.

Further information
Birmingham Children's Hospital NHS Trust http://www.bch.org.uk/ departments/clinicalchemistry/mcadd.htm.

Cystic fibrosis

CF is another autosomal recessive genetic disease inherited from carrier parents. It is currently not curable, although the search is on for gene therapy. CF affects the glands that produce body fluids or secretions. In CF these secretions are stickier and thicker than normal, affecting the lungs and digestive system. Common problems that people with CF experience include recurrent and severe chest infections, malabsorption and failure to thrive, diabetes, liver failure and infertility in males.

Early diagnosis of pre-symptomatic babies can prevent or reduce long-term damage from infection and other complications. Interventions include high-energy foods, enzyme supplements, and vitamin and mineral supplements to help a person with CF to get the nutrients he or she needs. Regular exercise is important to keep the body fit and healthy. Daily physiotherapy and breathing exercises help to keep the body healthy and prevent excessive build-up of mucus in the lungs. Antibiotics and other medicines are used to control lung infections and inflammation. If respiratory failure occurs, a lung transplant may be necessary. Early interventions may increase survival from the current median age of 31 years.

About 10–15% of children with CF will present soon after birth with meconium ileus causing bowel obstruction because the faeces are so sticky. When this occurs testing for CF must be done after the life-threatening complication is dealt with (Box 6.5).

Box 6.5 Key messages: cystic fibrosis

- CF is an autosomal recessive genetic condition that affects 1 in 2500 babies in the UK.
- Sticky mucus secretions cause digestive problems, recurrent chest infections leading to lung damage, poor growth and development.
- Some babies will require a second blood sample at approximately 21 days for further testing.
- Affected babies are seen by a specialist and started on treatment by 30 days of age.
- Screening may identify some CF carriers but is not designed to pick up all carriers, unlike the SCDs programme.

Further information
Cystic Fibrosis Trust http://www.cftrust.org.uk/
Screening brief: Neonatal screening for cystic fibrosis. *Journal of Medical Screening* **8**, 51, 2001.

Taking newborn blood spot samples

Midwives need to understand how laboratories handle blood spot samples to ensure that the samples they take are of good quality and will not be rejected. Repeating blood spots for no clinical reason other than an inadequate or contaminated sample distresses parents, the baby and the midwife concerned. The laboratories need to take standard-sized samples from blood spot cards with an exact amount of blood so that the metabolite or hormone measurements are accurate. The laboratories achieve this by punching holes using a 3-mm diameter automated punch, so the effect is rather like using an apple corer to take a sample of the centre of an apple. Good quality blood spots help the laboratory staff to provide a good and rapid service for families.

Keeping the baby's foot warm is a prerequisite for taking a good sample, as this ensures that blood will flow more freely. You may want to ask parents to ensure that the baby has socks on prior to the visit at which a blood spot is taken. Washing the baby's foot with warm water and drying it thoroughly will also warm the foot and prevent cooling through evaporation and dilution of the blood sample.

Midwives universally agree that the best way to soothe a baby to take a blood spot is to let it breastfeed, and that the midwife's best friend in taking blood spots is gravity. Midwives suggest several ways of producing this effect, for example letting the feet dangle over the edge of the mother's lap whilst breastfeeding. As the blood spot will need to be quite large before it drops, this position produces blood spots that are of adequate width, so that the laboratory staff are not searching for a small part of the card soaked through to the back. Squeezing the heel to encourage blood flow may damage the tissues sufficiently to alter the blood spot with plasma produced in response to the pressure and therefore affects the screening results (Box 6.6).

Box 6.6 Practice point

Problems are caused if:

- The heel is squeezed to produce a blood sample, as this forces tissue fluid into the blood and dilutes it.
- The specimen on the card is too small as there will be insufficient blood to test. This sometimes occurs because the midwife does not wait long enough for a large drop to form, it takes about 15 seconds for a good drop to form, waiting longer than 15 seconds will cause the blood to start clotting and also produce analytical problems.
- The card is smeared with several small spots (multi-spotting) within each circle. There will not be sufficient blood for punching 3-mm samples or for analysis.
- The sample is made up of layers of blood where drops of blood have been dropped on top of each other. This will give false positive results as the levels of metabolites or hormones being measured will be twice or thrice depending on how many drops have been placed on top of each other.
- There is incomplete saturation where the blood does not go through to the back of the card as there will be too little blood at the bottom of the sample. It is important to let the drop of blood fall onto the card. Pressing the heel vigorously unto the blood spot card compresses the fibres in the card and prevents the blood from soaking through to the back of the card.
- If the sample is contaminated or diluted from additives in the sample, for example water when the heel has not been dried after washing, or there is heparin from an arterial line in a neonate.

There do appear to be differences between types of blood spot lancet in achieving good samples (Shepherd et al., 2006), and many maternity units find that the cost of using slightly more expensive lancets is more than offset by the reduction in home visits to obtain repeat samples.

Babies on neonatal units, including preterm babies, will often have blood taken for reasons other than newborn screening. To reduce stress to the baby, parents and staff, blood for screening can be taken with other blood tests provided that no additives such as heparin get into the blood spot sample. A venous sample can be taken with a needle and syringe and can be dropped onto the card providing no intravenous infusions are being infused through that vein which may contaminate the sample.

Newborn hearing screening programme

The Infant Distraction Test (IDT), introduced in the 1960s, tests a child's reaction to sound, i.e. how it behaves, rather than the hearing pathway itself. It cannot be used effectively with children under 6 months of age and is not a sensitive or specific screening test. Evidence suggests that early identification of a child's hearing loss and early intervention improves the chances that the child will develop better language skills, and enjoy benefits in speech, social and emotional development (Davis et al., 1997; Crockett et al., 2005).

Studies from the USA (Yoshinaga-Itano et al., 1998, 2000) suggest that children will benefit if their hearing impairment is identified and appropriate intervention introduced by 6 months of age. Early identification also prevents the depressing and demoralising trawl round health visitors, GPs and hospitals to find out why there is no obvious reason that a child is not meeting developmental milestones.

Dissatisfaction with IDTs and technological improvements in screening led to a Health Technology Assessment (Davis et al., 1997), which showed that new, harmless and minimally invasive tests could cost-effectively screen a baby's hearing within a few hours of birth. The UK NSC set up a gradually rolled out National Hearing Screening Programme (NHSP) in 2001. Since May 2005, all new parents in England have been offered newborn hearing screening for their baby.

The majority of the programmes are offered before the baby is discharged from the maternity unit with community 'catch-up' clinics for babies who miss screening in hospital or those babies born at home. Some PCTs (mainly in rural areas) have commissioned community-based services, either in local clinics or at home. There is evidence from the screening programme that in hospital-based programmes there are high rates of non-attendance at catch-up community clinics so it is vital that as many babies as possible are tested in hospital. Some maternity units run in-house baby discharge clinics so that mothers do not have to wait on the post-natal ward for a health professional to screen their baby's hearing and then discharge them.

The screening programme picks up both unilateral and bilateral hearing loss. Although a baby with poor hearing in one ear can compensate with the ear that does function, children with one-sided hearing loss may have difficulty hearing sounds directed towards their ear with the hearing loss, telling which direction a sound is coming from, understanding speech when there is a lot of background noise and understanding quiet voices or soft sounds. Children with a unilateral hearing loss need to take extra care when crossing the road, as they may not be aware of which direction traffic is coming from if they cannot see moving vehicles.

Two simple screening methods are now used to screen babies by testing whether the hearing pathway is intact: automated otoacoustic emissions (AOAE) and automated auditory brainstem response (AABR).

Automated otoacoustic emissions

The AOAE test is quick and gives the result immediately. It works on the principle that a healthy cochlea will produce a faint echo when stimulated with a clicking sound. The screener places a small ear-piece, containing a speaker and a microphone, in the baby's ear. A clicking sound is played and if the baby can hear, the hair cells within the cochlea produce an 'echo' sound in response to this stimulus, which is picked up by the microphone in the earpiece, decoded and recorded on a computer. If the test records strong responses from the baby's ear, this tells the screener and parents that the baby has satisfactory hearing. It can be difficult to get a response if the baby is unsettled at the time of the test, if the room is noisy or if there is any residual fluid in the ear from the birth process. If the baby does not respond, the AOAE can be repeated after a few hours or an AABR can be done, as AOAE is never a diagnostic test.

Automated auditory brainstem response

The AABR screening test works by recording brain activity in response to sounds. Sound travels through the outer ear as vibrations. When it reaches the cochlea it is converted into an electrical signal. This travels along the auditory nerve to the brain where it is 'converted' into recognisable sounds. A series of clicking sounds are played through headphones that cover the baby's ears. Three small sensors connected to the computer equipment are placed on the baby's head to collect the electrical response in the auditory nerve and brainstem when the sound is transmitted to the brain. If the baby hears normally, the computer will report strong responses. If there is no strong response then the computer will report that a referral should be made. Babies that have been cared for in special or intensive care units will undergo both tests.

Unfortunately, no screen is 100% specific or sensitive, i.e. always identifies every case and never refers healthy cases. Babies may also develop hearing loss at any time in infancy. So, even if a baby has had clear responses following the hearing screen, it is good practice to give parents a checklist enabling them to identify the sounds a baby should be making and their reaction to sound at different stages of their development (Box 6.7).

Box 6.7 Key messages: newborn hearing screening

- 1.3 babies out of every 1000 births have a permanent hearing loss from birth.
- Newborn hearing screening should be offered to parents of all babies and should be completed by 4 weeks of age for well babies in hospital-based programmes and by 5 weeks of age for babies in community-based programmes. Babies cared for in special or intensive care for more than 48 hours should finish the screening process by 44 weeks' gestational age.
- Hearing screeners test babies by using automated otoacoustic emissions (AOAE) and automated auditory brainstem response (AABR) tests.
- The vast majority of all babies screened will show strong responses after the AOAE screening test. About 15% will be referred for the AABR screening test. If both screens indicate a possible hearing loss, whether in one ear or both, the screener refers the baby to the appropriate Audiology Department for diagnostic testing. About 3% of babies need a diagnostic test.
- Midwives should encourage all mothers to have their baby tested before being discharged from hospital as the non-attendance rate at community catch-up clinics is high.

Further information
Newborn Hearing Screening Programme website http://www.nhsp.info/index.php
Screening brief: Screening infants for congenital deafness. *Journal of Medical Screening*.

Newborn and 6–8-week infant physical examination

Everyone, including parents, agrees that it is helpful if every baby is examined carefully shortly after birth and again at 6–8 weeks to ensure that there are no obvious potential problems (Box 6.8). The examination should be by a health professional who has had supervised training in the systematic examination of babies. The examination should include overall physical condition, including jaundice, with specific attention to examining the eyes, heart, hips and testes where applicable.

> **Box 6.8 Key message: newborn and 6–8 week infant physical examination**
>
> Examination of newborn babies must be done by a health professional who has undertaken specific supervised training. A tool kit for training is available on the Internet.
>
> **Further information**
> http://www.nipetoolbox.screening.nhs.uk/toolbox/

Information giving and consent

Midwives are crucial in ensuring that women/parents have adequate and appropriate information at a level they can understand in order to make a decision about having their baby screened. Parents do have the choice of accepting screening for all or some conditions but midwives need to ensure that parents understand that newborn screening is recommended by health professionals and the DH and that it is based on the best evidence available. A midwife should ensure that the benefits of screening are clearly explained to the parents so that if they decline screening they are fully aware of the possible implications. This may have an impact on how they respond to signs and symptoms of disease in their unscreened baby and they may have a lower threshold for seeking help.

When discussing any screening test, the midwife can take the following logical steps to ensure that the information the women/parents receive is comprehensive:

- Determine woman's/parents' knowledge of the conditions being screened for.
- Explain that screening is recommended.
- Check understanding of screening versus diagnosis.
- Describe screening test offered locally, how it is done and the timing of the test.
- Explain the likelihood of a positive result.
- Explain and agree how and when results will be given.
- Explain that confirmatory/repeat testing may occasionally be required.
- Discuss the meaning and implications of the possible test result, including the implications for other family members in the event of a positive test result.
- Record the woman's/parents' decisions.

It is very rare for parents to decline newborn screening but when this occurs the midwife needs to explore the reasons and rationale behind that decision. It is possible that the decision to decline screening is based on misinformation and misconceptions, which can easily be resolved with appropriate information and explanation (Box 6.9). However, if parents make an informed decision to decline screening the midwife needs to take the action shown in the box for blood spot screening.

Box 6.9 If screening is declined

If the parent(s) decline screening for their baby, either for specific conditions or the full programme:

- The blood spot screening card should be clearly marked 'DECLINE' (and sent to the laboratory in the normal way. This enables the decline to be noted in the laboratory and passed on to the Child Health Records Department for recording.
- The health professional should ensure that the parents have full information on who to contact and how, should they change their mind.
- It is important that both the family GP and health visitor are informed of the decline in writing by the head of midwifery as this information may be of clinical importance in the future care of the child (UK Newborn Screening Programmes, 2005).

All newborn blood spots are retained in a safe and confidential place for a minimum of 5 years as part of quality management. This allows investigation of very rare failure to diagnose an affected child through screening by re-testing the original blood spots. Residual newborn blood spots may also be used for testing at the request of the child's doctor acting on behalf of the family, should the baby or another family member become ill. They can also be used for audit, training, improvement and development of laboratory methods relevant to screening, public health monitoring and other uses as allowed under the provisions of the Human Tissue Act (Great Britain, 2004: Section 55). There remains some confusion amongst health professionals as to whether babies are screened for HIV infection. HIV in babies is monitored by the Health Protection Agency (HPA) through their unlinked anonymous prevalence monitoring programme. This uses samples of blood left over from specimens taken for clinical tests, such as blood spot cards. The HPA requests random samples of cards from different geographical areas to look at prevalence in different parts of the UK. All specimens have patient identifying details permanently removed before testing. Individual test results cannot be linked in any way to the source patient. The programme surveys populations of specimens, not individual patients (HPA, 2002) and a positive sample cannot be traced back to a specific baby.

Residual newborn blood spots may also be used for research where the samples have been anonymised and the research project has ethical approval, as outlined in the Human Tissue Act (Great Britain, 2004) and in MRC Guidance (number 56, 2001) without individual informed consent. Very occasionally, research may involve contacting parents or their children, inviting them to take part. In these circumstances, parents and/or their children will be informed about this research and allowed time to decide whether or not to accept such an invitation. At the time of the initial blood spot sample, parents may choose not to be contacted with such future invitations. All research projects should have been approved by an ethics committee and be subject to peer review to ensure that the research is of high quality (UK Newborn Screening Programmes, 2005).

Pregnant women are now targeted with a plethora of information about many different things, including screening. It can be very difficult for women/parents to discern what screening they can access through the NHS and when. Women and their partners can often feel overwhelmed by the sheer wealth of information.

Timelines

The NSC has produced a timeline, a useful visual guide for both health professionals and women, which indicates optimal timing for screening for each of the antenatal and newborn screening programmes (NSC, 2006b) (Figure 6.1). We know from work done by the hearing screening programme that women want the information staggered so that they can consider information about newborn screening at the most relevant time and women say this is from about 28 weeks of pregnancy (Clemens et al., 2000; Sancho, 2006). It is therefore important that midwives act as a catalyst at this time by targeting women/parents with information at this stage. Midwives should examine care pathways and working patterns, and ensure this is an integral part of care.

Language

We need to ensure that parents understand all the complex messages listed above. Problems may be further compounded when parents do not speak English. The UK Newborn Screening Programme Centre (UKNSPC) and the NHSP have both produced patient information leaflets in several different languages to assist health professionals in discussing screening. These information leaflets aim to aid the consultation rather than replace it. Discussion with the health professional provides parents with the opportunity to ask for clarification and seek any further information they may need to make an informed choice (UK Newborn Screening Programmes, 2006; NHS Newborn Hearing Screening Programme, 2006).

Women/parents who do not speak English and need interpreters to translate screening choices can be a challenge for midwives. Sandall et al. (2001) showed in her study in East London that variations in uptake rates of Down's syndrome screening (31% Bangladeshi women, 67%

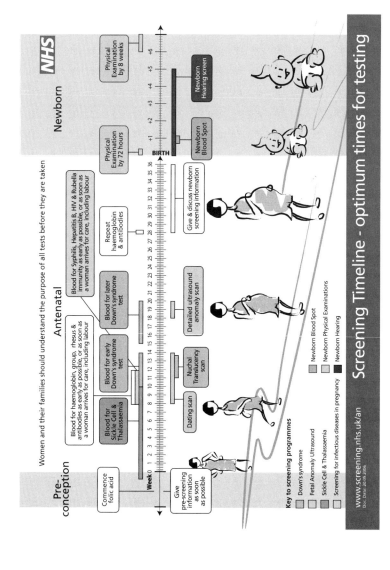

Fiugre 6.1 NSC screening timeline (http://www.screening.nhs.uk/cpd/timeline.htm). Reproduced with permission from the National Screening Committee.

African Caribbean women and 85% Caucasian women) were directly related to ethnicity and had a direct correlation to fluency in English.

The London region screening team has explored ways to help midwives in this area. In addition to searching the literature for good practice, we held a workshop in 2005. The delegates were a mixture of local antenatal screening coordinators (all of who were midwives), interpreters and healthcare advocates across London. The collaborative working and the poignant messages that came out of the day have influenced practice across the region in a very positive way. The 'take home' messages from the workshop are summarised in Box 6.10.

Box 6.10 Summary of important messages and points to consider when working with interpreters

Establish clear boundaries and expectations

- Brief the interpreter before the consultation so they know its purpose: taking a history, explaining screening results, breaking bad news, etc.
- Check whether the interpreter has time limits on the consultation, for example an appointment with another client elsewhere in the hospital.
- Establish rules of confidentiality: who will be told what about the consultation. The woman must be aware that everything she discloses to the interpreter will be passed on the healthcare professional and that the interpreter will only translate but will not give advice other than that given by the healthcare professional.
- Establish clear boundaries between the midwife and the interpreter and explain these to the woman and her family.
- Be conscious of the dynamics of the consultation, for example seating arrangements.
- Address the woman, not the interpreter.
- For interpreters: make women aware that some professionals may be quiet/silent when performing the test but will explain their findings later in the consultation.

Training which instills confidence
- Include interpreters in local training programmes and/or steering groups as appropriate.

Work collaboratively
- The clinician and the interpreter must view themselves as a team working collaboratively to achieve a specific goal, i.e. consider themselves equals allied together to accomplish what neither can do alone.
- Ensure interpreters are aware of departmental policy and local resources to support informed decision making, for example patient information leaflets.

Making the best use of health advocates and interpreters
http://careerfocus.bmjjournals.com/cgi/content/full/325/7355/S9a.

Improving screening by ensuring blood spots are taken on time

For certain conditions, like PKU and CHT, it is extremely important that screening is performed at the right time, ideally by day 5 (where date of birth is counted as day 0). Appropriate treatment and/or interventions must be commenced by day 21 in order to avoid irreversible damage.

Midwives across England have traditionally counted the baby's date of birth as day 1 if the baby is born before 12 noon and day 0 if the baby is born after 12 noon. This does not appear to be based on any evidence or documented guidance.

The Royal College of Midwives librarian searched archives dating back to 1937 and no record of this universal practice could be found. Experienced midwifery practitioners and scholars think that this practice started as a result of reporting bed states, which in the past were done at 12 noon. This provides a useful indicator for midwifery tasks such as weighing the baby and removal of sutures where appropriate and more importantly today for discharge planning, but midwives now need to change their method of counting to identify the date of birth as day 0, whatever the time of birth.

The UK Newborn Screening Programme Centre (UKNSPC) was established in 2002 with the overall objective of assuring high-quality screening services for babies and their parents and has produced six standards to underpin the quality assurance programme for newborn blood spot screening – Standard 1 relates to timely sample collection (Box 6.11).

Box 6.11 Standard 1

http://www.ich.ucl.ac.uk/newborn/download/policies_standards.pdf

Core Standard: 95% of first samples taken 5–8 days after birth (ideally on day 5).
Developmental Standard: 100% of first samples taken 5–8 days after birth (ideally on day 5) where the date of birth is counted as day 0 irrespective of the time of birth.

Taking the sample too early increases the chance of a false positive result for CHT due to the surge in thyroid stimulating hormone (TSH) immediately post birth. The consequences are that the baby may be subjected to a repeat test. Taking the sample late will mean a delay in critical treatment for a screen positive baby.

Current practice has improved generally since the publication of the national standards. In South-East London we have seen the rate of late samples (those taken on or after day 9) reduce from 6.4 to 4.9%. However, we are finding that the discrepancies in the way midwives in practice and the UKNSPC count the baby's date of birth are affecting the timing of blood spot sampling. This means that national standards are not being achieved and, more importantly, there is an impact on the clinical outcome of babies who are screen positive.

Great Ormond Street Newborn Screening Laboratory recently published data in its annual report of 2005–2006 showing a wide variation by hospital in samples that were taken too early (1.39–40.92% of samples taken prior to day 5).

Risks associated with newborn blood spot screening

There are various professional groups and stages involved in newborn blood spot screening. If and when errors occur they can impact on the next stage of the process and ultimately on the outcome for the child. Case studies 6.1 to 6.6 are real examples of incidents notified to the London screening team. We hope that these case studies will stimulate you to think about your individual practice and also about systems in your locality. Where these systems are not robust you may want to discuss the issues with your manager and ensure that everybody involved understands the inherent risks and the possible outcomes. Boxes 6.12 to 6.14 summarise the important lessons to be learnt from these cases.

Case study 6.1

Sample A took 23 working days to process as no *date of sample collection* was recorded on the card. This missing information was requested by the laboratory and was only provided 29 days later.

Case study 6.2

Sample B took 34 working days to process as no *date of birth* was recorded on the card. Despite an earlier request for this missing information, no correspondence was received by the laboratory. It was only after we wrote to the Director of Public Health that the missing information was provided 45 days later.

Case study 6.3

Sample C took 44 working days to process as the blood spot sample was taken too early at 3 days and therefore a repeat sample was requested. No response was received despite further reminders.

Case study 6.4

A blood spot sample was received by the laboratory on day 71 and appeared to have been taken on day 36. The laboratory immediately sent a letter to the midwifery unit asking for a repeat sample and investigation of the delay. It transpired that a student midwife had completed the first card and the sample had been taken on day 5 but the date of birth had been recorded incorrectly.

Box 6.12 Lessons to learn (1)

- Midwives need to ensure accurate documentation in all boxes on the blood spot card in the absence of bar coded labels. Laboratories need this information to check that blood spots have been taken within the correct time frame and in order to analyse and interpret their findings appropriately.
- Student midwives must be adequately supervised and the midwife mentor is ultimately accountable for the care given.

Case study 6.5

- A baby had a blood spot sample taken on day 5 but the midwife forgot to send it. When she realised this she took a repeat sample on day 87. The sample was received in the laboratory on day 90 and a result was issued on day 91 which showed a borderline result of CHT, so the blood spot was repeated on day 92. This was a human error and the midwife did disclose her error as soon as she found the card.

Box 6.13 Lessons to learn (2)

- Midwives and maternity units should develop individual systems for checking that samples are sent to the laboratory within 24 hours of sampling.
- Avoid keeping samples in handbags or briefcases. It is a good idea to have a special plastic food box for transporting each sample back to base or to post box.

Case study 6.6

A mother who is a health professional asked her health visitor for the result of the blood spot screen taken on day 5. The health visitor said 'No news is good news' but the mother was not happy with this response, and telephoned the UKNSPC. The UKNSPC contacted the laboratory and could not find a blood spot sample or result for this baby.

Box 6.14 Lessons to learn (3)

- Maternity units need systems in place to ensure that samples sent to the laboratory are received by the laboratory.
- Health visitors are responsible for ensuring that parents receive their baby's results, even if negative, between 6 and 8 weeks postnatally.
- Midwives should inform parents of this and encourage women to ask the health visitor at the postnatal visit.
- Robust child health systems are required to ensure that all babies under 1 year have a result or a 'decline screening' recorded.

Summary

It is hoped that you will now agree that this chapter is an essential read for community midwives and all those involved in newborn screening programmes. It is timely that maternity services address the issues raised, in advance of the further expansion of the newborn screening agenda.

Key points

- A good screening test is part of a comprehensive screening programme.
- Midwives have a duty of care to ensure that parents are fully informed of the implications of screening in order to maximise the benefits and minimise harm.
- Good technique is vital in collecting blood spot samples for newborn screening.
- In relation to the timing of blood spot screening, it is imperative to change the method of counting to identify the date of birth as day 0, whatever the time of birth.
- Midwives must ensure that they possess a sound knowledge of the newborn screening programmes in place, and keep abreast of the changes that will occur, in order to deliver evidence-based midwifery care fit for the 21st century.

References

Abramsky, L. (2003) *Prenatal Diagnosis – The Human Side* (eds L. Abramsky and J. Chapple), 2nd edn. Nelson Thornes, Cheltenham.

Clemens, C.J., Davis, S.A. and Bailey, A.R. (2000) The 'false positive' in universal newborn hearing screening. *Pediatrics*, **106** (1), 7–11.

Cochrane, A.L. and Holland, W.W. (1971) Validation of screening procedures. *British Medical Bulletin*, **27**, 3.

Crockett, R., Baker, H., Uus, K., Bamford, J. and Marteau, T. (2005) Maternal anxiety and satisfaction following infant hearing screening: a comparison of the health visitor distraction test and newborn hearing screening. *Journal of Medical Screening*, **12** (2), 78–82.

Cuckle, H.S. and Wald, N.J. (1984) Principles of screening. In: *Antenatal and Neonatal Screening* (ed. N.J. Wald). Oxford University Press, Oxford.

Davis, A., Bamford, J., Wilson, I., Ramkalawan, T., Forshaw, M. and Wright, S. (1997) A critical review of the role of neonatal hearing screening in the detection of congenital hearing impairment. *Health Technology Assessment*, **1** (10), 177.

DH (2000) Second Report of the UK National Screening Committee, Department of Health, London. http://www.nsc.nhs.uk/pdfs/secondreport.pdf (accessed December 2006).

DH (2003) Tackling health inequalities: a programme for action, Department of Health, London. http://www.dh.gov.uk/PolicyAndGuidance/ HealthAndSocialCareTopics/HealthInequalities/ProgramForAction/ ProgramForActionGeneralArticle/fs/en?CONTENT_ID=4072948&chk= %2B0wc2o (accessed December 2006).

Great Britain (2004) *Human Tissue Act 2004 (c30)*. http://www.opsi.gov.uk/ acts/acts2004/20040030.htm (accessed January 2007).

HPA (2002) *Prevalence of HIV and Hepatitis Infections in the United Kingdom: Annual report of the unlinked anonymous prevalence monitoring programme.* Health Protection Agency, London.

NHS Newborn Hearing Screening Programme (2006) Parent zone: information leaflet translations. http://www.nhsp.info/nhsphomeparent.php (accessed January 2007).

NHS Sickle Cell and Thalassaemia Screening Programme (2003) Antenatal screening policy. http://www.sickleandthal.org.uk/antenatal.htm (accessed January 2007).

NSC (2006a) Mission of the National Screening Committee. http://www. library.nhs.uk/screening/ (accessed January 2007).

NSC (2006b) NSC Screening Timeline. http://www.screening.nhs.uk/cpd/ timeline.htm (accessed January 2007).

Mezey, G.C. and Bewley, S. (1997) Domestic violence and pregnancy. *British Journal of Obstetrics and Gynaecology*, **104**, 528–531.

Reidpath, D. and Allotey, P. (2003) Infant mortality rates as an indicator of population health. *Journal of Epidemiology and Community Health*, **57**, 344–346.

Sancho, J. (2006) *Consultation with Midwives*. NHS Newborn Screening Programme, London.

Sandall, J., Grellier, R., Ahmed, S. and Savage, W. (2001) Women's access, knowledge and beliefs around prenatal screening in East London. http:// www.kcl.ac.uk/teares/nmvc/research/project/docs/77-THHT_Finalrept. doc (accessed January 2007).

Shepherd, A.J., Glenesk, A., Niven, C.A. and Mackenzie, J. (2006) A Scottish study of heel-prick blood sampling in newborn babies. *Midwifery*, **22**, 158–168.

UK Newborn Screening Programmes (2005) Newborn blood spot screening in the UK. Policies and standards. http://www.ich.ucl.ac.uk/newborn/download/policies_standards.pdf (accessed January 2007).

UK Newborn Screening Programmes (2006) Resources: parent information, parent leaflets. http://www.newbornscreening-bloodspot.org.uk/ (accessed January 2007).

Wilson, J.M.C. and Jungner, G. (1968) *Principles and practice of screening for disease*. Public Health Papers: No. 34, WHO, Geneva.

Yoshinaga-Itano, C., Coulter, D., Thomson, V. (2000) The Colorado Newborn Hearing Screening Project: effects on speech and language development for children with hearing loss. *Journal of Perinatology*, **20** (8) (Pt 2), S132–S137.

Yoshinaga-Itano, C., Sedey, A.L., Coulter, D.K., Mehl, A.L. (1998) Language of early- and later-identified children with hearing loss. *Pediatrics*, **102** (5), 1161–1171.

Breastfeeding and the role of the community midwife

Caroline Payne

Midwives spend a relatively brief amount of time supporting women during their pregnancy, birth and postnatal experiences. It is such a special time, but a woman has to make many decisions that have the potential to impact upon her and her child's life. One major decision is how to feed her baby.

Health education and health promotion are integral to the role of the midwife, and midwives working in the community have a key part to play in promoting breastfeeding as a means of improving public health overall. Whilst acknowledging that women must exercise choice, there is a wealth of evidence to support the statement that breastfeeding promotes health and formula feeding is related to ill-health.

This chapter presumes that the reader has knowledge of the anatomy of the breast, the physiology of lactation and the principles for good positioning and attachment. The aim is to explore the role of the community midwife in supporting the initiation and duration of breastfeeding. It will review the process associated with achieving Baby Friendly Initiative (BFI) status before moving on to present case studies for specific situations where additional expertise and intensive breastfeeding support might be needed.

Breastfeeding and health

Formula feeding is an adequate way of feeding a baby, but breastfeeding is best.

A key study of 545 children in Dundee took a longitudinal approach to link the choice of infant feeding to health outcomes during childhood (Wilson et al., 1998). Data relating to episodes of respiratory illness, growth, body composition and blood pressure was collected from birth to the age of 7 years and analysed in relation to the choice of infant feeding and the introduction of solids. Wilson et al. (1998) concluded that exclusive breastfeeding significantly reduces the incidence of respiratory illness and that exclusive formula feeding is associated with higher systolic blood pressures in childhood. The early introduction of weaning before 15 weeks of age was also linked to higher indices of body fat and weight in childhood.

Health is a continuum that can be influenced by sociological and political factors. One example that shaped attitudes towards breastfeeding in the UK was the introduction of subsidised formula milk at the end of World War II, as part of the welfare foods scheme. With good intention, the government of the day condoned the ready availability of subsidised formula milk. This coincided with a large increase in the number of women having their babies in hospital, where strictly regimented feeding schedules worked against the establishment of successful breastfeeding to a great extent. Dykes (2006) has explored the impact and the wider issues arising from the medicalisation of breastfeeding within the institutional setting of the hospital, to illuminate the steady decline of breastfeeding rates in the UK in the latter half of the 20th century.

The effect of this decline upon the nation's health is now emerging. It is well documented that formula feeding is associated with increased risks for infants of gastroenteritis, respiratory infections, otitis media, urinary infections, atopic disease (in families where there is a history), necrotising enterocolitis, obesity and diabetes.

Obesity and its link to type 2 diabetes, heart disease, hypertension and cancer poses a major threat to children. Dewey's (2003) literature review on the preventative effects of breastfeeding concluded that epidemiological evidence supports the fact that it is associated with a moderate reduction in the risk of childhood obesity. Some theories that might explain this effect include the following:

- Breastfeeding maintains normoglycaemia. In comparison, formula-fed babies have higher circulating insulin concentrations due to the greater protein content of formula milk. In theory, this encourages greater deposition of fat stores (Owen et al., 2006).
- Breastfeeding favours the development of appetite regulation. The changing nature of the composition of breast milk results in a higher fat content as the feed progresses, to act as a physiological message that tells the infant that he or she is 'full'. The composition of formula milk is constant and a formula-fed baby is reliant on his or her carer to regulate the volume of milk at each feed (IBFAN, 2004).

Nutrition in infancy has a life-long impact. An obese child is very likely to become an obese adult (Committee on Nutrition, 2003). This realisation must drive strategies aiming to tackle obesity in the future with clear recognition that breastfeeding promotes health. In the USA, Homer and Simpson (2007) urge a collaborative approach whereby policy makers, health providers and community groups work together to reduce rates of childhood obesity. Their interesting mnemonic ('BB210') puts breastfeeding first to underpin a summary of their overall strategy (Box 7.1).

Box 7.1 BB210

Breastfeeding

Body-mass index

2   fewer than 2 hours of television watching each day
1   more than 1 hour of physical activity each day
0   zero sugar-sweetened beverages

Homer and Simpson (2007)

Breastfeeding also offers recently identified health gains for women, including decreased risks of breast cancer, ovarian cancer and osteoporosis (Furber and Thomson, 2006). Dermer's (2001) review of the benefits of breastfeeding for women warns that related studies may have flaws in their design because definitions of breastfeeding can be inconsistent. She concludes that there is an estimated 11–25% reduction in the risk of breast cancer if a woman breastfeeds for 6–24 months and this timescale is cumulative across the period of reproduction. This is backed up by Jernstrom et al. (2004), who agree that increasing the duration of breastfeeding reduces risk. Their study focused on women carrying the breast cancer genes BRCA1 and BRCA2 to discover that if women carrying the BRCA1 mutation breastfeed for more than 12 months their risk for breast cancer is lower than those who have never breastfed.

The World Health Organization (WHO) recognised the superiority of breastfeeding and its benefits for health when they introduced a supportive international policy some time ago (WHO, 1981). Evidence underpinning such key policy has traditionally been focused on scientific evaluation of the constituents of breast milk. Morse (1992) suggested that this is concurrent with a medicalised approach that is of little value when seeking to improve breastfeeding rates. She presents a sound argument for researching cross-cultural, anthropological and experiential perspectives to improve our understanding of the complex interactions that promote, support or undermine successful breastfeeding. Scientific facts contribute to the body of knowledge about breastfeeding but have little impact on public health in isolation. Community midwives are particularly well placed to work with available evidence and can make a difference by applying it within a social model of care. This is nothing new. Midwives have always been engaged in public health work. What is new is that the role of the midwife is being highlighted in the UK and targets have been set to increase breastfeeding rates year on year.

Choice

The desire to breastfeed is often shaped through observation of the experiences and exposure to the attitudes of close family members and friends (Hoddinott and Pill, 1999). The quality of a mother's own breastfeeding experience will undoubtedly shape the perceptions and beliefs of her daughters and sons. A supportive network of family and friends that view breastfeeding positively are highly significant when a woman makes her choice. Wagner et al. (2006) note from their study that 95% of women who had been breastfed by their mothers chose to initiate breastfeeding. This figure dropped to 50.9% for women who had not been breastfed themselves. Partners and peers were also found to be extremely influential. Women were much more likely to breastfeed if their partners had been breastfed and viewed breastfeeding positively.

Initiation of breastfeeding

The DH in the UK undertakes a National Infant Feeding Survey every 5 years. Data from 2000 show that 71% of women in England and Wales chose to start breastfeeding. However, there are demographic factors associated with the initiation of breastfeeding that indicate a number of inequalities. For example, women employed in managerial and professional roles are much more likely to initiate breastfeeding (86%) than women who have never worked (54%). The woman least likely to initiate breastfeeding is generally young, belongs to a socially disadvantaged group and has poor educational attainment (Hamlyn et al., 2002). Under the NHS plan (DH, 2004b), the DH aims to reduce health inequalities and the goal set for breastfeeding rates is an increase of 2% each year. The focus on disadvantaged groups is being maintained through building upon the work of Sure Start initiatives nationwide. A more diverse approach towards breastfeeding education and support, from peers as well as professionals, is emerging (DH, 2004a).

Detailed data collected for the initiation of breastfeeding from 2003 to 2006 is available on the DH website. Here, you can identify individual rates and trends for each PCT. The good news is that the preliminary report for the 2005 National Infant Feeding Survey indicates an overwhelming rise for the initiation of breastfeeding in the UK (Bolling, 2006). In all four countries there were increases in all age groups, with one exception in the under 20s. In Scotland and Northern Ireland, this was particularly low with rates of 40 and 35% respectively.

Role of the midwife

The community midwife's role in promoting the initiation of breast-feeding starts with discussion at the booking visit (Box 7.2). The topic of infant feeding should also be revisited later on in the pregnancy. When a woman indicates that she does want to breastfeed it is impor-tant to make sure that she has access to any available educational and supportive resources. It has been identified that the use of more than one mode for communicating information increases the likelihood of good understanding (Kerr et al., 2005). The DH (2004b) has produced a beautifully illustrated leaflet called simply *Breastfeeding*. Paper copies are free on request and it is also downloadable in 11 languages: Arabic, Bengali, Chinese, Farsi, French, Gujarati, Kurdish, Punjabi, Somali, Turkish and Urdu.

Box 7.2 Practice point

- It is recommended that you talk about the advantages of breastfeeding for women and their babies before you ask a woman about her feeding intention.
- If you ask about her intention right at the start of the conversation, and she replies that her mind is made up to use formula milk, it then makes it really difficult to discuss breastfeeding.

Encourage women who want to breastfeed to attend antenatal breastfeeding sessions. Partners and grandparents need be made welcome too because they are the people who are going to support the woman and they need evidence-based information if myths about breastfeeding are going to be dispelled. If your community has post-natal breastfeeding support groups, it is a great idea to refer pregnant women to them. The more they learn in the antenatal period from women who are breastfeeding, the more confident they will feel when their baby arrives. They will also have an opportunity to tap into a supportive social network that they can return to after the birth.

Community midwives must support informed choice to enable parents to decide on the method of infant feeding that is right for them, but this does not mean that they cannot explore the reasons why women arrive at a particular decision (Box 7.3). It might appear unlikely that this opportunity for discussion will change the woman's chosen method of feeding but it is important to explore attitudes and dispel any misconceptions. Some women will change their minds. Wickham and Davies (2005) discuss the role of the midwife in empowering women through antenatal education. They recount how one midwife's adult-centred approach in facilitating an infant feeding session allowed prospective parents to identify the advantages and disadvantages of both feeding methods for themselves through group work. Each group then fed back to initiate a discussion and share insights. One woman thanked the midwife at the end of the session and demonstrated its effectiveness. The client-led format of the session had allowed the woman to reframe her original perceptions of breastfeeding as a difficult and potentially unachievable choice for her. As a result, she felt much more confident and had decided to breastfeed.

Box 7.3 Self-assessment point

- Do I offer unbiased information that supports choice?
- Do I have the skills to empower women to explore the available evidence effectively?
- Am I aware of available resources to support a woman's choice to breastfeed?

Duration of breastfeeding

It is good news that the rates for initiation of breastfeeding are increasing but if you look more closely at the National Infant Feeding Survey you will find that the definition of the incidence breastfeeding has remained unchanged since 1975:

> 'Incidence of breastfeeding is defined as the proportion of babies who were breastfed initially. This includes all babies who were put to the breast at all, even if this was on one occasion only.'
> Bolling (2006)

Data collected over time for the survey in 2000 illustrate the prevalence and duration of breastfeeding. This did not increase in England, but it has improved significantly in Scotland since the previous report. The definition used to assess the prevalence of breastfeeding is all inclusive. It encompasses exclusive breastfeeding, mixed breast and formula feeding and the accompanying introduction of solids. Hamlyn et al. (2002) illustrate the rapid fall in breastfeeding rates during the first year:

- 2 weeks   52%
- 6 weeks   42%
- 4 months   28%

- 6 months   21%
- 9 months   13%

Data from the 2005 survey should be made generally available in 2007 to illustrate that there has been some attempt to separate out prevalence figures according to whether breastfeeding was exclusive or mixed. Prevalence rates for exclusive breastfeeding at 6 months are negligible (BFI, 2007a). Merewood et al. (2005) agree that a standard definition for exclusive breastfeeding can only improve the reliability of data collected. This is an important point in light of the WHO's (2002) recommendation that exclusive breastfeeding for the first 6 months offers the best start in life for all infants.

Increasing the duration of breastfeeding is therefore a key priority for health professionals and the effectiveness of evidence-based midwifery care in the puerperium could readily be measured against the prevalence of continued breastfeeding. Factors that support continued breastfeeding are similar to those influencing its initiation. The three key reasons why women discontinue breastfeeding have been listed as:

- baby not latching on
- sore or cracked nipples
- woman perceives that the milk supply is insufficient.

(Dykes, 2006: 44)

Scott et al.'s (2006) Australian study emphasises that the duration of breastfeeding is negatively influenced if the woman experiences difficulty with breastfeeding in the first 4 weeks. They also explore the link between the introduction of pacifiers (dummies) for breastfed infants and the discontinuation of breastfeeding, to suggest that more research needs to be carried out. They question whether pacifiers are a cause of breastfeeding difficulties and postulate that they may be used in an attempt to alleviate problems.

All three of the key reasons for stopping breastfeeding relate directly to the remit of the midwife, but the task of improving breastfeeding rates is huge. Individuals play their part but a strategic intervention that fosters a team approach is much more likely to impact significantly. This is the rationale for discussing the BFI prior to looking at the role of the community midwife in supporting women with specific breastfeeding problems.

Baby Friendly Initiative

This worldwide initiative is led by the United Nations International Children's Fund (UNICEF) in collaboration with the WHO. Since 1991 it has been working to promote and support breastfeeding on a global scale. Utilising a strategic approach, the BFI works to ensure high standards of care for pregnant and breastfeeding women and their babies. They offer an assessment and accreditation pathway to reward successful institutions with full BFI status. Scotland is leading the way in the UK. Their devolved government has a breastfeeding policy, the Scottish Parliament is breastfeeding friendly and there is a breastfeeding lead in government. Almost 60% of all babies born in Scotland are born in hospitals holding BFI status, as opposed to only 10.4% in England (BFI, 2007b). Scotland's highly proactive and multifaceted approach towards breastfeeding has resulted in measurable improvements.

The UK BFI encompasses education, advice and audit to improve support for breastfeeding within the NHS. Healthcare providers are encouraged to adopt recognised best practice standards. These standards aim to ensure that all parents are able to make informed decisions about feeding their babies and then subsequently experience high quality, evidence-based support. The standards are well known as the 10 steps to successful breastfeeding (Box 7.4).

Box 7.4 10 steps to successful breastfeeding for the maternity services

1. Have a written breastfeeding policy that is routinely communicated to staff.
2. Train all healthcare staff in the skills necessary to implement the breastfeeding policy.
3. Inform all pregnant women about the benefits and management of breastfeeding.
4. Help mothers initiate breastfeeding soon after birth.
5. Show mothers how to breastfeed and how to maintain lactation even if they are separated from their babies.
6. Give newborn infants no food or drink other than breast milk, unless medically indicated.
7. Practise rooming-in, allowing mothers and infants to remain together 24 hours a day.
8. Encourage breastfeeding on demand.
9. Give no artificial teats or dummies to breastfeeding infants.
10. Foster the establishment of breastfeeding support groups and refer mothers to them on discharge from the hospital or clinic.

Vallenas and Savage-King (1997)

The 10 steps are supplemented by a seven-point plan for the protection, promotion and support of breastfeeding in community healthcare settings (Box 7.5). The first three points reiterate those of the 10-point plan. The focus then moves naturally to identify the importance of supporting women to maintain and encourage exclusive breastfeeding, with timely introduction of complementary solid foods. The remaining two points encompass the importance of a supportive community in the provision of a welcoming atmosphere in family friendly venues, and good co-operation between professionals, support groups and the community as a whole.

Box 7.5 Seven-point plan for the protection, promotion and support of breastfeeding in community healthcare settings

1. Have a written breastfeeding policy that is routinely communicated to staff.
2. Train all staff involved in the care of mothers and babies in the skills necessary to implement the policy.
3. Inform all pregnant women about the benefits and management of breastfeeding.
4. Support mothers to initiate and maintain breastfeeding.
5. Encourage exclusive and continued breastfeeding, with appropriately timed introduction of complementary foods.
6. Provide a welcoming atmosphere for breastfeeding families.
7. Promote co-operation between healthcare staff, breastfeeding support groups and the local community.

Vallenas and Savage-King (1997)

Working towards accreditation

Achieving BFI status requires long-term commitment to a staged process that has to be completed within 5 years. The initial step, whereby interested parties register a statement of intent with UNICEF, is simple and free of charge. The 'statement of intent' then triggers an action planning visit by a Baby Friendly advisor. The advisor supports staff in the development of an action plan that incorporates the needs of the local population. Within 12 months of the action planning visit, the healthcare provider must finalise the action plan and indicate that it has an evidence-based breastfeeding policy in place that satisfies BFI standards. It is then possible for UNICEF to award a Certificate of Commitment.

Within the following 4 years, there are three assessments to complete. The Stage 1 assessment examines the supporting framework that will enable implementation of the standards. Assessors scrutinise programmes of education for staff, and education programmes and supportive materials for pregnant and breastfeeding women. They will also want to ascertain that there are plans for recording the dissemination of evidence-based information to women and their families, and measures in place to audit practice effectively.

Preparation for the Stage 2 assessment revolves around the implementation and development of the educational programme for all staff. Theoretical components of the programme will be linked to observations of the clinical staff who are supporting breastfeeding in practice. The level of staff expertise is then audited to provide evidence that an appropriate level of knowledge and skills has been attained prior to the assessment taking place. This is then confirmed by the assessors, who will interview clinicians to satisfy themselves that Stage 2 has been achieved.

The final Stage 3 assessment is concerned with the effective implementation of the 10 steps for successful breastfeeding and the seven-point plan. Achievement of the standards will be supported by continuing audit and assessors will visit to speak to pregnant and breastfeeding women to assess their views about the quality of the service provision.

Full accreditation is an indication of excellent teamwork and a commitment to evidence-based practice. Accreditation remains current for 2 years, after which a reassessment is required to maintain ongoing Baby Friendly status. UNICEF and the BFI are non-profit making concerns but they do levy charges for accreditation to meet their expenses. From January 2007 the cost of the action planning visit plus the three assessments is quoted as £7030, but this may vary according to the size of the healthcare organisation.

It could be said that BFI accreditation represents the gold standard (or even the Holy Grail!) for breastfeeding. In the UK, the proportion of babies breastfed at birth increases by more than an average of 10% over a 4-year period in a BFI accredited hospital (BFI, 2007b). Internationally, babies born in BFI hospitals are seven times more likely to be exclusively breastfeeding at the age of 3 months, and 12 times more likely at 6 months. This carries huge implications for improvements in infant health. The subsequent reduction in hospital admissions for gastroenteritis and other medical conditions will soon recoup the initial financial outlay associated with acquiring BFI status if a broad and long-term view is taken (Box 7.6).

Box 7.6 Self-assessment point

- My trust has not yet signed up to the BFI – what am I going to do to actively promote the idea?
- Are neighbouring trusts signed up to the BFI?

Why aren't all trusts 'baby friendly'?

In light of the current economic climate, it is apparent that a large number of services are competing for a share of scarce resources. However, a short-term view that fails to identify the sustainable health benefits of the BFI ignores the significant impact that it can have upon public health, and also the public purse, for years to come. The National Institute for Clinical Excellence (NICE, 2006) has assessed the cost savings, in health terms, associated with going baby friendly. They looked at gastroenteritis, asthma and middle ear infection to conclude that a 10% increase in breastfeeding rates over 4–5 years will result in significant monetary savings for the NHS. This report only takes three illnesses into account but there are many more health benefits for both women and babies. It goes without saying that the human cost, for parents, of the emotional work associated with the hospitalisation of a child is immense.

The true savings for the NHS could be huge if we were to make a corporate leap to acknowledge the benefits of exclusive breastfeeding for 6 months or longer.

Nationwide initiatives to improve the diet and lifestyle of the nation are currently aiming to address issues such as heart disease, obesity and the prevention of type 2 diabetes. The Healthy Start programme has been implemented and the five-a-day campaign is now firmly embedded in a large part of the nation's consciousness. But the loop will be incomplete unless healthcare organisations support comprehensive achievement of Baby Friendly status or similar initiatives. NICE (2006) recommends the adoption of an externally validated tool, such as the BFI, as a minimum standard. One can't help wondering whether this vital recommendation could be backed up by a short-term, centrally funded financial commitment. Such an investment would pay for itself many times over in monetary as well as health terms.

Back to basics

Good positioning and attachment are vital elements for successful breastfeeding. They are often referred to in the same breath but it is important to differentiate these two components. Positioning refers to both the woman and the baby. The woman needs to be comfortable and aware of a range of positions that she might try. Attachment is viewed as a skill that the woman has to master. The baby's instinctive reflexes will elicit the 'wide gape' and that moment needs to be seized to bring him or her onto the breast effectively. The traditional positions for breastfeeding have evolved over time but Colson (2005) suggests that there are alternatives. Her concept of biological nurturing encourages a more holistic view of breastfeeding within the context of 'a two-person, whole body experience' where the woman should be free to choose the position that is most natural for her and the baby. If these two people are relaxed, comfortable, and take time to enjoy skin to skin contact with the baby in a prone position, he or she will very often attach to the nipple spontaneously. Colson's work challenges long-held professional perceptions of the ways in which breastfeeding should be facilitated and must be considered in light of the failure to significantly improve the duration of breastfeeding to date (Box 7.7).

Box 7.7 Self-assessment point

- Am I confident that I have the skills to teach women how to position and attach a baby at the breast?
- Do I need to update my skills by attending an evidence-based workshop?

If we backtrack to the reasons why women discontinue breastfeeding, the biggest negative influence was cited as 'problems during the first 4 weeks'. Many of these early breastfeeding problems arise directly from poor positioning and attachment. This reinforces the need for all practitioners to maintain and develop their expertise in breastfeeding support. Effective intervention should support the woman, alleviate the problem and result in the continuation of breastfeeding.

When problems with breastfeeding are encountered, it is vital to take a look at the whole picture. This involves three steps: history taking, listening to the woman's concerns and observation of a breastfeed.

History taking

Community midwives frequently have to tackle breastfeeding problems after the woman's discharge from hospital. It is important to explore what has been happening since that first feed and the time spent taking a history will pay dividends. A history can offer a number of clues to help you work out the underlying cause of the problem and inform solutions. If the woman does not speak your language, you will need to access the services of an interpreter.

History taking can be informal but it is usually more constructive to use a formal checklist and make notes as the discussion progresses. A record of the history can then be retained with the postnatal record to support good practice in contemporaneous documentation.

A good starting point is an assessment of the family and social support available to the woman. Finding out about the attitude of partners, grandmothers and friends is particularly important. Many women have worries about family members or older children and their reaction to the new baby. If a woman has very little social support it might be appropriate to refer her to other agencies. We know that breastfeeding duration is closely linked to the timing of a woman's return to work. This might be a factor that is worrying her, so enquire about her plans and whether her employer is supportive of breastfeeding women. She might also have related financial concerns on her mind.

Ask about the woman's general health before pregnancy and currently. Does she have any medical conditions such as diabetes, epilepsy or thyroid disorder? She may have anxieties about prescription medicines or be concerned that her intake of caffeine, alcohol, nicotine or non-prescription/recreational drugs is affecting the baby via her breast milk. Does she have a physical disability or any learning difficulties? Has she ever had breast surgery or is she worried about any physical changes in her breasts?

Pregnancy is the next logical topic. Try to find out if this was a low- or high-risk pregnancy and the uptake of antenatal care. If the woman did not have antenatal care she will have missed out on opportunities to find out more about breastfeeding from discussion with a midwife, available literature and participation in antenatal breastfeeding preparation sessions.

Next, review what happened during labour and around the birth and check on the gestational age. Kroeger and Smith (2004) have explored the relationship between birth practices and their impact upon breastfeeding. They identify many thought-provoking issues, including the fact that maternal and fetal hormonal stressors during a long second stage of labour can significantly delay the first feed. Epidurals and associated anaesthetic agents have also been linked to breastfeeding problems in the first 24 hours, notably in relation to poor attachment (Baumgardner et al., 2003). This offers a rationale for finding out about the length of labour and type of pain relief used.

Find out whether or not the baby had unhurried skin-to-skin contact immediately after the birth. Did he or she go to the breast for an early feed and was help and support offered by attendants?

Postnatal care will hopefully have incorporated 'rooming-in' so the majority of women will be able to tell you about the quality and quantity of early feeds. Ask about the support that the woman received and dispel any concerns relating to conflicting advice through reference to available evidence. If any supplementary feeds were given to the baby, find out the reasons why. Determine whether the feeds were expressed breast milk or formula and how they were offered, i.e. by bottle, cup, syringe or spoon.

Transitional care facilities have reduced the need to separate mothers from babies who need close observation but there will always be a number of infants who spend their first few days of life in special care or neonatal intensive care units. If the woman and her baby were separated, she should have been shown how to express her breasts by hand, or with a pump, to initiate and maintain lactation.

Information about the health of the baby needs to include gestational age, birth weight and the trend of weight gain or loss. Is the baby a singleton? If he or she is one of multiples then ascertain his or her birth order. What was the baby's condition at birth and did he or she receive any drugs or require resuscitation? Vigorous oropharyngeal suctioning of the neonate can confuse the innate reflexes governing sucking and swallowing mechanisms to disrupt the 'suck–swallow–breathe' pattern essential for effective breastfeeding (Kroeger and Smith, 2004). Find out whether the baby experienced any birth trauma and if he or she was admitted to the special care or neonatal intensive care unit.

A healthy baby will be passing urine approximately six times in a 24-hour period and wet nappies should be full and heavy. Look at the nappy to see if it contains the telltale 'brick dust' deposits indicative of concentrated urates and note the colour and consistency of the stool.

Information relating to the feeding pattern and behaviour should identify whether the baby wakes himself or herself to root for a feed, and the frequency and length of feeds. Ask the woman if one breast is sufficient at each feed and whether the baby detaches spontaneously then settles. If the baby has been vomiting, find out the nature of the vomitus and ask whether or not it is projectile.

A physical examination of the baby should follow your history taking. You need to make sure that this is a well baby. Differentiate between physiological and pathological jaundice, look for signs of infection in the cord, eyes and nail beds, assess tone and irritability, examine the mouth and buttocks for signs of thrush, and look at the anterior fontanelle to assess hydration.

Listening, and observing a feed

Give the woman time to talk about the problems she has currently. Use open questions, listen actively and always be sensitive. Breastfeeding is tied in to many emotions, including the fear of failure and guilt. If breastfeeding is painful, you need to explore the nature of the pain to discover when it began and what type of pain it is. Does it occur before, during or after a feed and how long does it last? Pinpoint the location of pain. It might be in the nipple, the breast or even the uterus. Find out whether the woman has used a dummy, nipple shields/protectors or breast shells, and if so, for how long.

Ask about the support that other health professionals have given, reiterate good advice and check whether anybody has observed a breastfeed before. Once you have taken the history, ascertained that the baby is well and identified the woman's concerns the next crucial step is to observe a breastfeed.

In order to diagnose the problem, and decide on the most appropriate advice to offer, you will need to observe the whole feed from beginning to end. Look at the shape of the woman's nipple and observe her position, and that of the baby, as she attaches her baby at the breast. Ask how it feels because many women have been told that breastfeeding will hurt and they expect it to be painful. Unless you ask about discomfort or pain specifically, some women will not disclose it. When the baby detaches at the end of the feed it is vital to observe the nipple again. It should be the same shape as it was when the feed started.

Breastfeeding case studies

It is impossible to offer a comprehensive guide to all breastfeeding problems here but Case studies 7.1 to 7.3 have been chosen to illustrate the use of the framework described in the previous section – history taking, listening, and observing a feed. These case studies also address topical issues that community midwives will be familiar with in day-to-day practice (see Boxes 7.8 to 7.10). The names of the individuals concerned have been changed to preserve their anonymity.

Case study 7.1

Ankyloglossia

Wendy is 29 and has just had her second baby. She used non-pharmacological support measures in labour and had a spontaneous vaginal birth. Sally, the community midwife, made her first home visit when baby Abby was 2 days old. She was aware that Wendy had breastfed her first baby very successfully for 8 months and asked how it was going this time. Wendy said that she was quite concerned because Abby was 'fussing' at the breast and kept coming on and off. This had made Wendy's nipples sore. Abby was rooting and looked hungry so Sally suggested to Wendy that it would be a good idea for her to assess the problem by observing how Abby fed.

Wendy made herself comfortable. She sat upright in a straight-backed chair and used a pillow to support Abby at a comfortable height on her lap. Sally watched as Wendy brought Abby to attach at the breast in a way that was instinctive to her. As Abby opened her mouth Sally noticed that the baby's tongue was heart shaped and did not appear to have the usual range of movement around the mouth. Sally said nothing at this point but continued to observe closely as Abby attached to the breast but kept slipping off repeatedly. Sally then suggested trying a different position. Wendy tried holding Abby in the 'underarm/rugby tackle' position but this didn't seem to improve the situation and Wendy's sore nipples were becoming more painful.

Continued

Sally asked to look inside the baby's mouth and she could see that Abby's tongue was anchored firmly by a tight frenulum, commonly referred to as a 'tongue tie' but known in the medical literature as ankyloglossia. Sally encouraged Wendy to have a look at the frenulum and the shape of Abby's tongue. Sally then gently explored the impact that ankyloglossia can have upon the initiation of breastfeeding. Wendy said that when Abby had been checked over in hospital by the paediatrician he had pointed the 'tongue tie' out but had said that it would not cause any problems. Sally explained that for many babies that is the case, but for Abby it was causing a problem because it was preventing her from breastfeeding effectively.

Wendy had access to the Internet at home and Sally helped her to locate and download some information about ankyloglossia from the NICE and Baby Friendly websites. Sally also contacted her colleague, the infant feeding specialist, who came to see Sally to undertake a further assessment. Once again, she observed how Abby fed to assess the impact of the ankyloglossia upon breastfeeding. The specialist then discussed the option of dividing the frenulum and listened to Wendy's opinions.

Wendy had already had time to look at the information available and the procedure and associated risks were discussed. She then made an informed decision to go ahead. The Baby Friendly website has a list of contact details for all of the medical practitioners in the UK who will perform division of the frenulum. The nearest practitioner was accessed via the clinical pathway in place in the ear, nose and throat department of the local district general hospital. An appointment was made for 3 days later.

Sally visited Wendy daily to support her with breastfeeding and manual expression in the days prior to the appointment. On the day after the procedure, Abby was feeding from the breast when Sally arrived. The pain had gone, Abby's attachment was sustained well and these best breastfeeds since the birth added up to a contented baby and a smiling Wendy.

Box 7.8 Practice point: ankyloglossia

- Ankyloglossia is associated with uncoordinated sucking, poor attachment and nipple trauma. Sequelae include cessation of breastfeeding, poor weight gain, dehydration and speech defects (Hall and Renfrew, 2005).
- Early referral to and assessment by lactation specialists is urged to prevent the development of intractable breastfeeding problems (Blenkinsop, 2003).
- NICE guidelines (2005) support the option of frenulotomy, in appropriate cases, by suitably trained practitioners.

Case study 7.2

Thrush and breastfeeding
Mary was breastfeeding her first baby, George, who was 2 weeks old. Mary had experienced sore nipples in the first few days but this had resolved with good support that had helped Mary to position and attach with a good technique. Other than that, breastfeeding had been going well. Mary had been visited daily by her community midwife because her blood pressure had been raised. She needed medication for this but it had been effective and was now controlled. The community midwife was visiting that day with a view to discharging Mary and George into the care of the health visitor.

When the community midwife arrived, she found that Mary and George had had an unsettled night and Mary was complaining of an intense pain in her breast after feeding. She had been massaging her breasts because she thought that she had been developing mastitis, and felt that this had made them more painful. Mary felt well otherwise and certainly had no flu-like symptoms. Her breasts were not engorged and there were no red patches across the skin of either breast.

The midwife observed a breastfeed. Mary had no pain during the feed but she did complain of nipple soreness at the end of it. Positioning and attachment were reviewed and the small adjustment of bringing George's body closer to Mary's did help to ease the soreness subsequently. The midwife looked inside George's mouth and noted that he had oral candidiasis. Mary had noticed some white spots in his mouth but had thought that it was just milk residue from previous feeds. The midwife suspected that Mary also had candidal infection in her milk ducts. She gave Mary the leaflet produced by the Breastfeeding Network called *Thrush and Breastfeeding* and advised her to make an urgent appointment with her GP to get a prescription for herself and the baby. Mary was also advised to take the leaflet with her to the appointment. The midwife telephoned Mary the next day to find out what the GP had suggested. He had confirmed the midwife's findings and prescribed the appropriate treatment.

Mary made a full recovery. She needed more support from the community midwife for a few days, as the treatment did take a couple of days before it was effective. Coupled with improved positioning and attachment, the nipple soreness resolved and breastfeeding became enjoyable again. Mary and George started to go to a community-based breastfeeding group for ongoing support.

Box 7.9 Practice point: candidiasis

- Explain to the woman that thrush thrives in moist, dark environments and offer advice on general hygiene, i.e. hand washing and changing towels.
- Dummies (and teats), if used, need to be sterilised using a hypochlorite solution, e.g. Milton, to destroy the yeast organism.
- Treatment for thrush should be topical and systemic – detailed prescribing information is available on the Breastfeeding Network website. To prevent re-infection, both the woman and the baby need to be treated, even if only one of them has symptoms.
- Thrush is frequently, but mistakenly, diagnosed when poor positioning and attachment are the cause of pain. The end result of this poor practice means that both women and their babies are exposed unnecessarily to prescription medication.
- It is always vital to assess positioning and attachment when women complain of any type of breast or nipple pain.

Case study 7.3

Social support and communication

Sophie is 16 years old and lives at home with her parents. They were initially less than supportive during her pregnancy but they are much more positive since the birth of baby Robbie. Sophie is very keen to breastfeed. She found out about the benefits of breastfeeding during a session at school about healthy living and parenting. Her parents are less keen on the idea of breastfeeding because they feel that bottle feeding would allow her family to help her more, and Sophie could also go back to school sooner. She has a friend called Jess who is a little bit older at 18. Jess is breastfeeding her own baby and gives Sophie some support, but she still finds things difficult at home sometimes, particularly when she is tired. Sophie has some literature about breastfeeding that the community midwife gave her and she has shared this with her parents, but they still keep harping on about using the bottle.

Sophie came home from hospital when Robbie was 2 days old. By day 4, she finds that she is spending most of her time in her bedroom because she feels embarrassed about breastfeeding in front of her dad and her brother who tend to make jokes about it. She has a strong character and usually copes with a ready and smart reply but is, unsurprisingly, starting to find their attitude tedious and irritating.

Sophie has sore nipples and has tried using some cream that her mother bought from the chemist. It didn't help at all so she then tried Jess's suggestion – expressing some milk and letting it dry on the nipple. This helped a little but the soreness is still there. Her nipples have been sore really since day 1. To begin with they were only sore at the start of a feed but now they are sore all the way through and it is making her feel miserable. There is no chair in her bedroom and she usually feeds Robbie whilst sitting on the bed.

Continued

The community midwife asks Sophie if she can observe how Robbie feeds and explains how doing this will help her to work out how to improve things. As Sophie prepares to feed her son she appears nervous and uncomfortable. The midwife senses this straightaway and starts to chat about everyday things and a TV programme that they both saw last night. This relaxes Sophie and the midwife asks whether she might like to try sitting in chair to feed because it might help improve her positioning. Sophie goes to speak to her dad and a few minutes later he brings a straight-backed chair into her bedroom. A couple of pillows help Sophie to get herself comfortable and she holds Robbie in the crook of her arm with his body facing away from her. The midwife notices some breastfeeding leaflets from the hospital on the bedside table. She uses the pictures in the leaflets to illustrate good and bad positioning for attachment and then sits with Sophie, guiding her verbally to move Robbie into different positions. Sophie and Robbie then achieve good attachment and a pain-free breastfeed. Robbie detaches himself after 40 minutes and looks very full and contented. Sophie says that she now feels that she understands the principles of good positioning and attachment.

Over the next 2 days, Sophie is visited by another community midwife and continues to gain confidence. The original midwife visits again several days later to find Sophie breastfeeding downstairs in the company of the rest of her family. Sophie is given details of a local breastfeeding support group in case she wants to go along to meet other mums – and perhaps she will share some tips with others on how to deal with parents who want you to formula feed!

Box 7.10 Practice point: social support and communication

- Always ask for permission to observe a breastfeed. Framing the request to state that you wish to 'watch how the baby feeds' is less threatening than stating that you want to 'watch the woman feed her baby' (BFI, undated).
- A hands-off approach to assisting with positioning and attachment seems to be the most effective. The woman learns by making mistakes – your role is to be there to correct these and guide her. Only if the woman is struggling, or does not understand you, should you help with hands on – aim to build confidence rather than undermine it.

Summary

There is no doubt that community midwives have a key role in promoting, supporting and sustaining breastfeeding. This chapter has explored that role to place it within the wider context of national guidance, targets and initiatives that aim to improve the public health of the nation. Exclusive breastfeeding for the first 6 months of life has been highlighted as the best possible start in life but there is a great deal of room for improvement in relation to figures for its duration in the UK. The BFI has been identified as one strategy that has proven results in relation to initiation and prevalence rates.

All midwives have a responsibility to update their skills in supporting women who choose to breastfeed and the case studies have highlighted examples of good practice at a clinical level. Individuals need to work together to ensure a proactive approach that incorporates a clear strategy, partnership within the wider community and the best available evidence.

Key points

- Breastfeeding promotes health.
- A woman's decision to breast or formula feed is heavily influenced by her partner, other close family members and her peers.
- The rates for initiation and prevalence for breastfeeding in the UK are improving, but the number of babies enjoying exclusive breastfeeding at 6 months is negligible.
- Initiatives such as BFI are recommended by NICE as strategies that support minimum standards of care for breastfeeding women and their babies.

Useful contacts: sources of support and information

National Childbirth Trust (NCT)
www.nct.org.uk

Association of Breastfeeding Mothers (ABM)
http://abm.me.uk

Breastfeeding Network
www.breastfeedingnetwork.org.uk

La Leche League (LLL)
www.lalecheleague.org

Baby Friendly Initiative
www.babyfriendly.org.uk

NICE Guidance re Ankyloglossia
www.nice.org.uk/IPG149

References

Baumgardner, D.J., Muehl, P., Fischer, M. and Pribbenow, B. (2003) Effect of labour epidural anesthesia on breastfeeding of healthy full-term newborns delivered vaginally. *Journal of the American Board of Family Practice*, **16** (1), 7–13.

BFI (undated) *Clinical Practice 1: Observing a breastfeed*.

BFI (2007a) The Infant Feeding Survey 2005; findings related to the Baby Friendly Initiative Baby Friendly News, Issue 24, July 2007, UNICEF UK. http://www.babyfriendly.org.uk/newsletter/news_0607.html.

BFI (2007b) Why do we need the baby friendly initiative? http://www.baby-friendly.org.uk/page.asp?page=17 (accessed March 2007).

Blenkinsop, A. (2003) A measure of success: audit of frenulotomy for infant feeding problems associated with tongue-tie. *MIDIRS Midwifery Digest*, **13** (3), 389–392.

Bolling, K. (2006) *Infant Feeding Survey 2005: Early Results*. The Information Centre, London.

Colson, S. (2005) Maternal breastfeeding positions: have we got it right? (2). *The Practising Midwife*, **8** (11), 29–32.

Committee on Nutrition (2003) Prevention of pediatric overweight and obesity. *Pediatrics*, **112**, 424–430.

Dermer, A. (2001) A well-kept secret: breastfeeding's benefits to mothers. *New Beginnings*, **18** (4), 124–127.

Dewey, K.G. (2003) Is breastfeeding protective against child obesity? *Journal of Human Lactation*, **19**, 9–18.

DH (2004a) *Good Practice in Innovation and Breastfeeding*. The Stationery Office, London.

DH (2004b) *Breastfeeding*. The Stationery Office, London.

Dykes, F. (2006) *Breastfeeding in Hospital: Mothers, Midwives and the Production Line*. Routledge, Oxford.

Furber, C.M. and Thomson, A.M. (2006) 'Breaking the rules' in baby-feeding practice in the UK: deviance and good practice? *Midwifery*, **22** (4), 365–376.

Hall, D. and Renfrew, M. (2005) Tongue tie. *Archives of Disease in Childhood*, **90**, 1211–1215.

Hamlyn, B., Brooker, S., Oleinikova, K. and Wands, S. (2002) *Infant Feeding, 2000: A survey conducted on behalf of the Department of Health, the Scottish Executive, the National Assembly for Wales and the Department of Health, Social Services and Public Safety in Northern Ireland*. The Stationery Office, London.

Hoddinott, P. and Pill, R. (1999) Nobody actually tells you: a study of infant feeding. *British Journal of Midwifery*, **7**, 558–565.

Homer, C. and Simpson, L.A. (2007) Childhood obesity: what's health care policy got to do with it? *Health Affairs*, **26** (2), 441–444.

IBFAN (2004) *Breastfeeding Briefs No 38: Breastfeeding, Childhood Obesity and the Prevention of Chronic Diseases*. International Baby Food Action Network.

Jernström, H., Lubinski, J., Lynch, H.T., Ghadirian, P., Neuhausen, S., Isaacs, C., Weber, B.L., Horsman, D., Rosen, B., Foulkes, W.D., Friedman, E., Gershoni-Baruch, R., Ainsworth, P. and Daly, M., Garber, J., Olsson, H., Sun, P., Narod, S.A. (2004) Breast-feeding and the risk of breast cancer in BRCA1 and BRCA2 mutation carriers. *Journal of the National Cancer Institute*, **96** (14), 1094–1098.

Kerr, J., Weitkunat, R. and Moretti, M. (2005) *ABC of Health Behaviour: A guide to successful disease prevention and health promotion*. Elsevier, Edinburgh.

Kroeger, M. and Smith, L. (2004) *Impact of Birthing Practices on Breastfeeding: Protecting the Mother and baby Continuum*. Jones and Bartlett, Massachusetts.

Merewood, A., Supriya, D.M., Chamberlain, L.B., Phillip, B.L. and Bauchner, H. (2005) Breastfeeding rates in US baby friendly hospitals: results of a national survey. *Pediatrics*, **116**, 628–634.

Morse, J. (1992) Euch, Those are for your husband!: examination of cultural values and assumptions associated with breast feeding. In: *Qualitative Health Research* (ed. J. Morse). Sage Publications, California, London, New Delhi.

NICE (2005) *Division of Ankyloglossia (Tongue-Tie) for Breastfeeding: Understanding NICE Guidance – Information for People Considering the Procedure for their Baby, and for the Public*. NICE, London.

NICE (2006) *Routine Postnatal Care of Women and their Babies: NICE Clinical Guideline no. 37*. NICE, London.

Owen, C.G., Martin, R.M., Whincup, P.H., Davey Smith, G. and Cook, D.G. (2006) Does breastfeeding influence risk of type 2 diabetes in later life? A quantitative analysis of published evidence. *American Journal of Clinical Nutrition*, **84**, 1043–1054.

Scott, J.A., Binns, C.W., Oddy, W.H. and Graham, K.I. (2006) Predictors of breastfeeding duration: evidence from a cohort study. *Pediatrics*, **117**, 646–655.

Vallenas, C. and Savage-King, F. (1997) *Evidence for the Ten Steps to Successful Breastfeeding*. WHO Child Health and Development Unit, Geneva.

Wagner, C.L., Wagner, M.T., Ebeling, M., Ghatman, K.G., Cohen, M. and Hulsey, T.C. (2006) The role of personality and other factors in a mother's decision to initiate breastfeeding. *Journal of Human Lactation*, **22** (16), 16–26.

WHO (1981) *International Code of Marketing of Breast Milk Substitutes*. World Health Organization, Geneva.

WHO (2002) *Global Strategy on Infant and Young Child Feeding*. 55th World Health Assembly, Geneva, World Health Organization.

Wickham, S. and Davies, L. (2005) Are midwives empowered enough to offer empowering education. In: *Birth and Parenting Skills: New Directions in Ante-Natal Education* (eds M. Nolan and J. Foster). Churchill Livingstone, Edinburgh.

Wilson, A., Forsyth, J.S., Greene, S.A., Irvine, L., Hau, C. and Howie, P.W. (1998) Relation of infant diet to childhood health: seven year follow up of cohort of children in Dundee infant feeding study. *British Medical Journal*, **316**, 21–25.

Safeguarding children

Judy Byrne

'Safeguarding children' is a term that has recently replaced the more familiar phrase of 'child protection'. Pearsall and Trumble (2002) define a child as a young human being who has not reached the age of discretion, and describe the concept of protection as 'keeping safe', 'defending' and 'guarding against danger, injury or disadvantage'. From these definitions, one can easily deduce the relevance of child protection to the role of the community midwife.

Protecting children is everyone's responsibility and this message has been firmly delivered through the findings and recommendations of Lord Laming's (2003) enquiry into the tragic death of Victoria Climbié. Following every serious case of child abuse or neglect there has been considerable consternation that greater progress has not been made to prevent such reoccurrences. Reviews and enquiries over the past three decades have consistently identified the same issues: poor communication and information sharing amongst professionals and agencies; inadequate training; poor support for staff and a failure to listen to children. Laming's enquiry was no different.

As midwives, it might be time to consider updating the term 'woman-centred care'. Replacing it with 'woman- and child-focused care' would reflect our concern for families as a whole. Midwives have been listed amongst a number of professional groups who have failed to identify the signs of serious abuse or make appropriate referrals (DH, 2002). Hospital midwives have an integral role in child protection and this must not be underestimated, but community midwives have a unique opportunity to observe many aspects of family life and children of all ages in their own homes. A midwife's role in safeguarding children is not limited to the unborn and neonates. It extends to all children that she or he comes into contact with. Practitioners must act at all times to identify and minimise risks for every child and have a duty to report any concerns to appropriate personnel (NMC, 2004a).

Reflecting on the involvement of midwives in the history of child protection, it can be said that midwives have led the way in statutory legislation. Supervisors of midwives were appointed with the introduction of the Midwives Act (Turner, 1902) and their prime concern has always been the protection of mothers and babies from harm. Legislation has developed over the past century and the current act no longer focuses only on the protection of babies from poorly trained midwives, but also on the protection of babies and children from harm caused by anyone. Supervisors of midwives must ensure that the needs of the woman and baby are the primary focus of their practice (NMC, 2004b).

The fact that child protection is becoming an integral part of a midwife's role could be seen as a poor reflection of 21st century society, but it may be that we are just getting better at identifying concern and taking action. Whatever the reason, it is clear that midwives are increasingly finding themselves involved with safeguarding issues. It is important to be vigilant because 1 in 10 households will experience child abuse in one form or another, and it often occurs in conjunction with the 1 in 4 households encountering domestic abuse issues (Great Britain, 2004a). All health professionals must also be alert to the possibility of a colleague causing harm to a child. Although the case of Beverley Allitt, a state enrolled nurse who murdered four children while they were inpatients on a hospital ward, is thankfully an exceptional scenario it must never be forgotten (Dyer, 1993).

Midwifery care aims to empower mothers and fathers to become loving and caring parents and it can be very difficult, emotionally, for midwives who are involved in safeguarding issues. No matter how experienced a midwife is, the safeguarding role is a daunting prospect due to its nature and complexity. This chapter is written for community midwives and also their hospital-based colleagues. It aims to offer practical guidance but will begin with a review of underpinning legislation. This will lead into the practicalities of safeguarding children, to include the identification of abuse, appropriate referral and management for midwives.

The Children Act (Great Britain, 1989)

To equip you with the basic knowledge to fulfil your important role in safeguarding children, it is necessary to have some understanding of the relevant legal framework. There are currently 25 700 children on the child protection register in England, most under the category of neglect. The child protection register is due for abolition in the very near future, as its usefulness is doubtful. It is being replaced by a system whereby children are safeguarded through child protection plans.

The protection of children is not new. The term 'battered baby' was first coined in the 1960s and this recognition of child abuse publicly challenged family life for the first time in history. It led to an increase in public awareness, particularly after the media publication surrounding the sad death of Maria Caldwell in 1973. Resulting legislation came into being in an attempt to reduce any further failings.

Box 8.1 Key landmarks

- **1976** The government advised that all local authorities should have a register of children at risk.
- **1989** The Children Act (Great Britain, 1989) came into force in 1991.

The Children Act (Great Britain, 1989) changed the threshold at which the state could intervene in family life. It introduced the concept of 'significant harm' and defined categories of abuse whilst focusing on the duties and responsibilities of parents, rather than their rights. The Act also proposed that professionals should work in partnership with parents, and recognised that children are best brought up within their own family. The duty to provide support to families was placed upon local authorities, but the Act also placed a statutory duty on health, education and other services to assist them in carrying out these duties. In practical terms this means that a midwife has a statutory duty to cooperate with social services in cases of child protection. You may hear this referred to as a section 47 enquiry.

Section 47 of The Children Act (Great Britain, 1989) requires local authorities to make such enquiries as they deem necessary (known as 'the Local Authority's duty to investigate') to enable them to decide whether they should take any action to safeguard a child's welfare. Such cases would include:

- a child who is the subject of a emergency protection order (EPO)
- a child in breach of a curfew order or in police protection
- a child thought to be in danger of significant harm.

Section 47 requires that you cooperate with the local authority during any enquiry into a child safeguarding issue. The Children Act (Great Britain, 1989) makes it lawful to apply for court orders pertaining to child protection concerns and these are explained below.

Emergency protection orders

EPOs are legislated by Section 44 of the Act. If a court is satisfied that there is reasonable cause to believe that a child is likely to suffer significant harm if he or she is not removed to accommodation provided by the applicant (i.e. the local authority), or if he or she does not remain in the place that they have been accommodated in, then the court can order an EPO. The order places the child under the protection of the local authority for a maximum period of 8 days and this can be extended for a further 7 days in exceptional cases. An EPO can be sought to prevent a parent taking a baby home from hospital where there are safeguarding concerns relating to a neonate. If parents resist in complying with an EPO then the police must be summoned. They will then forcibly remove the child from its parents. If a home birth is planned when there is an EPO in existence, the police and social services must be summoned by the community midwife before the birth is imminent.

Accurate and detailed information from the midwife may be required during application for an EPO. Anecdotally, there is often disagreement amongst midwives regarding the proposed actions in cases of an EPO because details are only known to a few necessary personnel and taking a baby from its newly delivered, reluctant and distressed mother can be viewed as extreme. There is no doubt that the situation is extremely distressing for all involved. It is worth noting here that the Human Rights Act (Great Britain, 1998) should also be considered. It confers children with the same rights as adults to guarantee that no-one be subjected to torture, degrading or inhuman treatment or punishment (Article 3). Article 8 of the Human Rights Act outlines the right to a private family life without interference, except in accordance with the law. In practical terms, if a midwife knows of, or suspects that, a child is at risk, as outlined in Article 3, then they must take action. There is no right of appeal against an EPO and further practical advice is given later in the chapter under advice for midwives surrounding safeguarding around the time of birth.

Child protection orders (Section 46)

The police can take a child into their protection if they believe the child to be at risk of significant harm and can act to prevent the removal of a child from hospital if they believe the baby to be at risk of such harm if he or she were removed. This power can be used if a baby's removal from hospital needs to be prevented because an EPO is not in place. The order only lasts for 72 hours and is instigated by phoning 999.

Care, supervision and child assessment orders

A care order places the child under the care of the local authority. The child does not have to live separately from its parent(s), but if a dispute ensues between the local authority and the parent(s) over arrangements for the child, the local authority will decide in the child's best interests. If a full care order cannot be obtained, due to time constraints or lack of time to collect information, an interim care order will be sought to give a local authority shared parental rights that parallel a care order.

A supervision order does not give the local authority shared parental responsibility, but it does provide a right of access to ensure the child's welfare. A supervision order can last up to 1 year but may be extended to 3. The local authority will always act in the best interests of the child and Section 37 of The Children Act offers further information.

Child assessment orders are granted by the courts (under Section 43) and may be used in non-emergency situations where parents do not cooperate with the authorities. One example might be when parents will not allow a medical assessment of their child. An application for a child assessment order would usually be made by a social worker and can be appealed against.

The Children Act (Great Britain, 2004b)

The government responded to the Laming enquiry with the Green Paper *Every Child Matters* (ECM) (DH, 2003). It provided overwhelming evidence of the need to improve outcomes for vulnerable children. The Children Act (Great Britain, 2004b) came into being to drive the implementation of the Green Paper's recommendations, starting with the creation of the post of a children's commissioner for England. The post-holder has a remit to promote awareness of the views and interests of children (commissioners were already established in Wales and Scotland). Part two of the Act is concerned with improving accountability for children's services within each local authority area, and local authorities are required to promote cooperation between the various agencies involved in safeguarding children. These include police authorities, local probation boards, strategic health authorities (SHAs) and PCTs.

Local safeguarding children's boards

Local safeguarding children's boards (LSCBs) are currently being set up across England to replace non-statutory area child protection committees. They will pave the way to abolish the child protection register and set up comprehensive information-sharing databases. The Children Act (Great Britain, 2004b) further promotes multidisciplinary working by specifying a requirement for some agencies (including PCTs and NHS trusts) to work together to make arrangements that safeguard and promote the interests of children. The membership of an LSCB includes a child protection midwife and nurse. The midwifery members of these boards feed relevant information back into the maternity services provided by the relevant NHS trust. Your NHS trust should have established hospital trust based safeguarding meetings where a child protection midwife will be a participant.

The actions set out in The Children Act (Great Britain, 2004b) are a direct response to attempt to address the failings highlighted by Lord Laming (2003). These can be summarised as:

- poor communication between professionals and agencies
- failings in the area of child protection training
- poor support for staff
- issues where the concept of confidentiality was misunderstood.

The Children Act (Great Britain, 2004b) does not replace or even amend much of the 1989 Act, but it does build on it to robustly and effectively underpin the ECM document. ECM is all about protecting and improving the life chances of all children. It aims to reduce inequalities to help children achieve what they deserve from life with its focus on four main areas:

- supporting parents and carers
- early intervention and effective protection
- accountability and litigation
- workforce reform.

It has responded to the issues of poor inter-agency communication and concerns about confidentiality through the introduction of information for professionals, supported by innovative new frameworks and tools. These include the common assessment framework (CAF), the lead professional role and mandatory training for all who come into contact with children through their professional role.

Working Together to Safeguard Children (Department for Education and Skills, 2006a) is a national framework document. It is a direct response to Lord Laming's (2003) request for a document that supports open inter-agency communication. It contains statutory guidance and non-statutory practice guidelines. The document is extensive and can be referred to in order to build upon the practical guidance outlined in this chapter (Box 8.2). It is intended for all organisations and individuals who work with children. A wealth of related information for professionals is available on the ECM website at http://www.everychildmatters.gov.uk (accessed May 2007).

Box 8.2 Key policy documents and resources arising from ECM

- The National Service Framework for children, young people and maternity services (DH, 2004).
- Sharing information: Practitioners' guide (Department for Education and Skills, 2006b).
- The Common Assessment Framework for children and young people: Practitioners' guide (Department for Education and Skills, 2006c).
- What to do if you are worried a child is being abused (Department for Education and Skills, 2006d).

Additional relevant legislation

Two additional pieces of legislation that are highly relevant to community midwifery practice are The Sexual Offences Act (Great Britain, 2003a) and The Female Genital Mutilation Act (Great Britain, 2003b).

Sexual activity under the age of 16 years is an offence and the Sexual Offences Act is clear that a child under the age of 13 years is not legally capable of consent. Midwives must be vigilant here and consider who the father of the baby is. All cases of pregnancy in girls under 16 years of age should be discussed in confidence with a named child protection midwife and/or a supervisor of midwives. Pregnancy in any girl under 13 years of age must be reported to the police.

Female genital mutilation (FGM) has been illegal in the UK since 1985. If relevant, FGM should be discussed during pregnancy to give women information relating to the legal and child protection issues in the UK. It is now an offence for UK nationals or permanent UK residents to aid to procure the procedure abroad or carry it out in another country, even if it is legal in that country. Midwives need to be aware that FGM is an offence in the UK because they may well witness the aftermath of the procedure in adults and possibly babies. The Act states that parents cannot remove any girl with UK nationality, or a permanent UK residence, to any place in the world to undergo FGM (Box 8.3).

Box 8.3 Practice point: female genital mutilation

- Alarm bells should be ringing if parents or carers tell you that a child is 'going away for a holiday'. It has been noted by Lee (2007) that Amsterdam is a centre for FGM.
- Any healthcare professional who is concerned that FGM is being considered has no choice but to report the matter urgently as a child protection issue.

Practicalities for midwives

For continuing professional development purposes, all staff working with children should attend training and regular updates in safeguarding and promoting the well-being of children. There are six levels of training, dependent upon your responsibilities and level of seniority. Every practising midwife must undertake level 1 and 2 child protection training, with the frequency of regular updates being determined locally. Supervisors of midwives, named child protection midwives and midwifery managers should receive level 3 training (Box 8.4).

Box 8.4 What is expected of you?

As a midwife you must be able to:

- understand the risk factors and recognise children in need of support or safeguarding
- recognise the needs of parents who may need extra help in bringing up their children and to know where to refer for advice and assistance
- recognise the signs of abuse to an unborn child
- contribute to enquiries from other professionals about children and their families or carers, e.g. children's social services
- liaise closely with other agencies, including other health professionals
- assess the needs of children and the capacity of parents/carers to meet the child's needs
- plan and respond to the needs of families, especially the vulnerable
- contribute to child protection conferences and strategy discussions
- contribute to planning and delivering support for children at risk of suffering, e.g. increased surveillance of parenting skills whilst in hospital and at home
- ensure access to support services, e.g. mental health services
- play an active part through the child protection plan in safeguarding children from significant harm
- provide ongoing support through proactive work with children, their families and expectant parents
- contribute to serious case reviews and their implementation, e.g. assistance in carrying out an EPO.

If you are the first health professional to identify concerns or problems you will undoubtedly question what action you should take, if any. Just remember that child protection is everybody's business and *never presume that someone else has already identified the problem* because they may not have done so. As a matter of urgency you must discuss your concerns with a relevant professional and, however difficult, make a referral if appropriate. If your actions can be founded at the time of the referral you will not be chastised if proved wrong. You do not owe a common law duty of care to parents but you do have a duty of care to the child (McMahon, 2005).

The nature of any concern and your intention to make a referral should ideally be discussed with parents before the referral is made. However, there are times when this is not possible. For example, if you believe this could put an unborn baby at risk of significant harm because the woman will go into hiding and no longer seek antenatal care, or if discussing your concerns regarding a child were to put your own safety at risk. If you do make a referral without parental knowledge then this must be made explicit to children's services along with your rationale for not discussing it with the parent(s).

Identifying vulnerable situations for children

Neglect and abuse are forms of maltreatment. Someone may abuse a child through inflicting harm or by failing to prevent it. Children may be abused by a known or unknown adult or another child. The context might well be within the family but it can also occur in an institutional or community setting. Abuse can be physical, emotional, sexual or actual neglect.

There is no definitive answer as to what constitutes abuse or neglect, but there are a number of signs that can alert you to possible child safeguarding issues. Midwives are continually observing women and unborn/newborn babies. This incorporates assessment of a family's well-being and can have a direct impact on children's and women's health. However, the identification of a vulnerable family does not necessarily require referral for child protection reasons. Some of the situations you may encounter will be made clearer if you discuss them with an appropriate professional who is experienced in child safeguarding issues (Box 8.5).

Box 8.5 Vulnerable families

Vulnerable families might include some of the following:

- families living with domestic abuse
- families dealing with substance misuse issues, including alcohol – these may not manifest until after the birth when a baby exhibits signs of neonatal abstinence syndrome.
- parent(s) with a known mental health diagnosis or learning difficulties
- those in low social economic groups
- women or men whose previous family/children no longer live with them – ask yourself why
- babies born to women who are unbooked and received no antenatal care, or those presenting at a hospital out of their normal area
- unplanned home births
- women living in temporary accommodation
- migrant families
- surrogate pregnancies.

Community midwives are often the first professional to discuss and/or identify issues of domestic abuse with a woman. Domestic abuse is now viewed as a child protection issue and taken very seriously. If a woman discloses the fact that she is living with an abusive partner, but does not want to pursue any help for herself or her unborn baby, she must be made aware that you have a professional duty to refer to children's services if there are concerns for the baby's welfare. The police now have dedicated teams dealing with domestic abuse. If they are called to an incident where there are children (born or unborn) living at the address, the local children's social services office and named health visitor will be informed automatically (Box 8.6).

Box 8.6 Practice point

Community midwives come into contact with vulnerable families on a daily basis. To aid decision making, consider asking yourself the following questions:

- What is the family's parenting capacity?
- Can the parents deliver basic needs of warmth and food?
- Can they ensure safety?
- Can they give emotional warmth and stimulation?
- Is there stability and consistency in their lives?

In cases of surrogacy, the biological mother retains her status as the mother in legal terms. If she is married and her husband was aware of the pregnancy then in law it is his baby, regardless of who provided the sperm. It is important to appreciate that a midwife's duty of care is for the pregnant woman and her child, not the couple who are expecting to take the baby home. Consent for any procedures or medication for the baby must be given by the biological mother. She cannot be forced into giving her baby up if she changes her mind. It is also noteworthy that parents obtaining a baby through surrogacy are not screened in the same manner as for adoptive parents (Great Britain, 1990).

Referral

As previously discussed, midwives may have concerns for other members of the family with whom they are working, i.e. older children, but for ease of use this section will relate to the unborn or newborn child.

If you have any safeguarding concerns when caring for a family at home or in hospital, you should check the case notes for any instructions relating to child protection issues. There may be an 'at risk' file kept on the labour ward, containing information pertaining to a child's safeguarding issues from out-of-area children's social services or other maternity service providers. You may initially learn about concerns from children's social services, or you may be the identifier of concerns (Box 8.7).

> **Box 8.7 Signs of abuse and/or neglect**
>
> - Neglect of basic needs, e.g. warmth and food.
> - Poor physical care, inadequate hygiene, inappropriate dress.
> - Emotional abuse, e.g. derogatory remarks about the child or baby: ugly, naughty, bullying, etc.
> - Fabrication of illness by parent/carer.
> - Grasp or bite marks, bruises, scalds, unexplained fractures.
> - Delay in seeking medical advice.
> - A torn frenulum.
> - Vague history, lacking detail and inconsistent.
> - Inappropriate parental reaction to an injury, for instance parents do not appear to care or be worried.
> - Unrealistic parental expectations, e.g. expecting baby to sleep all night.
> - Blaming child or baby unreasonably, e.g. soiled his/her nappy in order to irritate its parents.
> - Undermining comments, such as 'naughty baby', 'ugly baby'.

Documentation

Concern about a child's welfare should be recorded contemporaneously. Your records may be needed in future legal proceedings or for your own use in compiling a report for a strategy (discussion) meeting and/or child safeguarding conference. Your documentation must clearly distinguish between fact and fiction. You can record your judgement, as long as that judgement and subsequent related decisions made are clearly recorded as such. All records should be clear, concise, comprehensive and in plain English to enhance inter-agency communication.

Show caution if you are asked questions by anyone regarding safeguarding issues. Clarify why they are asking you and what the information will be used for; is it being documented? If so, ask for it to be read back to you – remember this information may be presented at a child safeguarding conference or as evidence in a criminal court, where it will be challenged and repeated many times. It must be accurate and true.

How to refer

In the first instance you can discuss concerns and gain confidential advice from a children's access centre, but it may not be appropriate to reveal the name of the family at this point. Children's services access centres are obliged to investigate your concerns if you identify the family. If time allows, or you are unsure of your actions, discuss your concerns with a named child protection midwife, nurse or supervisor of midwives. Do not hesitate to use the on-call midwifery managers or supervisors system in an emergency or out of hours. There should be agreed formats, developed by the local safeguarding board and its partners, for referral to local authority children's social care services. If you telephone your concern to children's social care services you must follow this up in writing (or by fax) within 48 hours. This initial written referral should be a multidisciplinary document, usually known as the Common Assessment Framework (CAF). A CAF offers a basis for early referral and information sharing between organisations. Confirmation of a referral should be sent to you within one working day of its receipt. If you do not receive this within 3 working days you must contact children's social services again (Department for Education and Skills, 2006a: 108).

Procedure following referral

If the family is already known to children's social services they may move straight to a strategy meeting to which you, as the midwife, will be invited. This meeting will decide whether the child is in need, or in need of protection. 'Children in need' are defined under Section 17 of the Children Act (Great Britain, 1989) as those whose vulnerability is such that they are unlikely to reach or maintain a satisfactory level of health or development without the provision of children's services. 'Children in need of protection' are at risk of suffering significant harm under Section 47 (Great Britain, 1989), i.e. a child deemed in need of protection (Box 8.8).

Box 8.8 Practice points: referral

- If concerns about the future care of an unborn baby child arise later than 30 weeks' gestation an urgent referral is appropriate.
- If you become aware of a pregnancy in a family where there have been previous child protection concerns, share this information promptly with children's services. Do not presume that they already know of this new pregnancy.
- When a social worker has concerns regarding an unborn baby they must share this information with the named midwife and midwifery services, especially if there are concerns about substance misuse or domestic abuse.
- Bear in mind that a definition of neglect includes the failure of a woman to attend any antenatal appointments.

If a family is not already known to children's social services, an initial assessment must be carried out within 7 days of the referral. The purpose of the initial assessment is to identify whether or not any services are required. Information will be gathered from all relevant parties, including the midwife. It may be that there are no concerns about the present or future care of the baby. If no further intervention is planned you should be informed of this outcome in writing. In cases where the need for further support has been identified the child will be classed as a child in need. If more serious concerns are identified and the child is at risk of significant harm, he or she will be deemed as a child in need of protection (Great Britain, 1989).

Child in need and a midwife's duty

An 'in need' plan must be prepared and distributed before a baby is born. The community midwife needs to remind other professionals involved that the plan must be in place well before the estimated date of delivery because babies often arrive before their due date! The plan should detail any extra support that needs to be put in place when the baby is born and must be shared with community and hospital midwives, health visitors and the named child protection midwife. If relevant, it should also be placed in the hospital case notes to ensure explicit instructions for staff whilst the baby is in hospital. It will include guidance to inform social services when the baby has been born. Owing to the difficulty associated with the assessment of parenting skills before the baby is born, it is necessary to direct the staff caring for the woman and her baby to assess and document their interactions after the baby is born. Any documentation relating to how a woman cares for her baby in the early days following the birth can be used to identify whether the family would benefit from additional sources of support. It might also be used at a later date in a court of law if further concerns arise and actions are taken.

Child in need of protection and a midwife's duty

When an initial assessment identifies that a baby is in need of protection before or after it is born, a core assessment will follow as a matter of course. The nurse consultant for child protection must be advised by children's social services that a core assessment is being undertaken and she should then inform all relevant professionals. As a midwife you will be asked to contribute any relevant information that you possess.

A core assessment informs the decision to proceed to a child protection conference where all health professionals with related information will be asked to attend. This includes the midwife and the future health visitor. The parent(s) will also be invited and are often in attendance whilst you give your findings. This can be very daunting if you are not prepared, but support and assistance are available if you feel that you need it. Child protection conferences need to be held as soon as possible so that the birth plan can be communicated well in advance of the event itself. It is good practice to have the plan in place by 32 weeks' gestation and, once again, the community midwife needs to remind the other agencies of the urgent need for this to be completed. A child protection conference should only take place after the 32nd week of a woman's pregnancy if the pregnancy has been concealed from health professionals.

Child protection birth plan

If the decision is that a child protection plan is required, this will be put together by the core group within 10 days of the child protection conference. Any infant who is the subject of a child in need of protection plan requires a hospital birth plan to ensure that all health professionals coming into contact with the newborn baby are aware of the plan and their role. In many areas it is the midwife's responsibility to ensure the hospital (or home) birth plan is communicated to the trust child protection midwife and relevant midwifery staff, and placed strategically in the hospital case notes. Birth plans for children in need of protection are formulated at the child protection conference and a pre-printed format is usually available for use. If a pre-printed version is not available you need to consider a number of points, summarised in Table 8.1.

The child protection conference must have representation from the maternity services to ensure that the above points are addressed, the plan secured in the case notes and relevant agencies informed.

The forcible removal of an infant from its mother may seem very harsh to the midwifery staff that have seen the woman give birth to, bond and breastfeed that little individual. But be reassured, this sort of separation is only recommended where there are serious concerns for the safety of the baby. A more usual scenario allows the mother to keep her baby with her, caring for him or her under the observation of the midwifery staff, coupled with detailed documentation and ongoing inter-agency cooperation.

When an EPO is in place and the baby is removed from its parent(s), he or she will subsequently be cared for in the neonatal unit for practical reasons of security. The baby will remain there for up to 48 hours unless medically required to stay longer. Suitable accommodation, usually with a foster mother, will then be arranged by social services.

Being involved in the removal of a baby from a mother is a very distressing event for all concerned. Parents will often give their baby to social workers voluntarily, but occasionally they do not and this situation is dreadful for all involved. In my own experience, it is clear

Table 8.1 Considerations regarding birth plan for a child in need of protection.

Questions	Considerations
When should children's services be contacted?	• Obtain relevant phone numbers for the named social worker and team leader, as well as the emergency 24-hour social services contact number. • If an EPO is in place, children's social services will need to be informed before the birth occurs. Do not wait – inform them as soon as the woman arrives in labour.
What level of contact can the parent(s) have with their baby after the birth?	• Define the level of supervision required precisely. • If the plan dictates that the baby needs constant supervision whilst in the care of the hospital, ask whether your unit can achieve this. • Constant supervision may or may not be feasible on a postnatal ward. If this degree of supervision is required then it must be discussed between the midwife and other agencies involved because constant supervision may only be possible if mother and baby are separated, i.e. baby nursed in the NICU with supervised access for the parent(s). In this scenario, supervised access should be provided by children's social services.
Who can have contact with the baby?	• Sometimes grandparents or the father of the baby are the initial or only concern and must therefore be denied access to visit the child in hospital or at home.
Can the mother/ parents take the baby home with them?	• Parents may try to discharge the baby against medical advice. You cannot stop them unless an EPO is in place. An EPO cannot be obtained before the birth, so there may be delay. • If necessary, a social worker can wake a magistrate and obtain an EPO out of office hours. • If an EPO is being sought and the parents are attempting to remove the baby from hospital, you are advised to delay the discharge or move the baby to a place of safety elsewhere in the hospital, but only if it is safe for you to do so. • Inform children's services and phone 999 immediately. The police will exercise their powers of judgement to remove the baby to a place of safety.
What if parents try to remove the baby when there is an EPO in place?	• Call 999 for assistance. The police will react quickly if you inform them, quoting the EPO number. Again, be aware of your own safety and do not put yourself or others in your care at risk of harm.
What can be done to minimise risk when there is a history of violence within this family?	• If there is any past history of violence within the family the police will share this information with relevant parties at the child protection conference. Parents will be excluded from this part of the meeting if circumstances dictate. • When it is deemed likely that there are concerns about violence you can request a police incident number and place it in the plan in a prominent place. This is not always suggested, so *if you are concerned you must be proactive*. When a police incident number is quoted by healthcare staff calling for assistance the response will be rapid and appropriate. Quoting the incident number allows immediate access to relevant information from police files.

that emotions amongst midwives are high and there is always a crucial need to discuss and debrief with all the staff involved.

Home birth and EPOs

Where a home birth is chosen and an EPO is to be obtained, then special precautions are needed, not only to protect the child but also the health professionals. A management of risk meeting must be convened where the police and an ambulance trust representative will be present to compile the plan for a birth at home. It will be necessary to have the police and social services on standby at the house whilst you are attending the labouring woman. The agreed management of risk strategy will be added to the birth plan and communicated as before.

It will be necessary for two midwives to be present at the house at all times throughout labour and the birth. The police will accompany the social worker to serve the EPO and remove the baby to hospital in the first instance. The police have powers to prevent the baby being taken away from the house before an EPO is obtained and it will be necessary for the midwives to stay at the house until after the baby is removed.

Once again, this is a very disconcerting scenario for midwives, at odds with their usual role of a woman's advocate. These decisions are not taken lightly and are only put into place if there is real concern for the baby's safety – the safety of the baby is uppermost in these cases. Help and support are available from your supervisor of midwives or manager in these difficult cases. Don't go it alone – asking for support is a sign of strength and insight rather than a sign of weakness.

Out of area

Some women choose to deliver in a unit other than their local maternity hospital. Where there are safeguarding concerns and/or a plan in place, it is imperative that this is shared with the unit designated for the place of birth. The midwife in attendance at multidisciplinary safeguarding meetings is charged with this role and must ensure that the relevant maternity services and hospital are provided with the relevant information as soon as possible.

If there are concerns regarding a baby born in your local unit whose mother lives in another local authority area, it is important that the relevant local children's services are alerted. However, any urgent protective measures can be carried out locally through referral to your own social services and police force. In a situation where concerns have been raised and the family moves out of the area, or if it is suspected that they may access maternity services elsewhere, then other areas will need to be informed nationwide. The children's social services team manager is responsible for alerting other children's services to these concerns and providing details. The named consultant nurse for child protection is responsible for informing all other maternity units of the concerns, details and contact numbers, in case the woman arrives unannounced and unbooked to give birth at an alternative unit.

Summary

When a child in need or a child in need of protection has been the subject of safeguarding measures during pregnancy and around the time of birth, a follow-up meeting will be arranged within 3 months of the baby's birth day. You will be invited to this meeting as the midwife concerned, and will probably find that the information you have to offer is limited in comparison to the other professionals in attendance. Despite this, it is a vital part of the role of the midwife. It can also be very valuable for you to find out how the ongoing situation is being managed and the results and progress made to date. Very often there is good news to report, but whatever the outcome it is likely that your participation will help you to rationalise the experience, place it in context and reflect.

As a midwife every contact you have with a pregnant woman provides an opportunity for you to support and engage with her. You are the professional she is most likely to forge a relationship with to share very personal and confidential information, such as mental health problems, domestic and sexual abuse and dependency on alcohol or drugs. These may be long-standing problems that she has been dealing with alone up until now. Pregnancy is a window of opportunity that can prompt a woman to reconsider her own and her child's safety. The privileged position of a community midwife provides a unique opportunity to engage with women, assess the family unit and possibly prevent family problems such as abuse of vulnerable children in the future.

Your role involves the recognition and appropriate referral of any concerns you have regarding the safeguarding of all children. This is a hugely challenging area and the related legislation is constantly changing. Midwives have a significant part to play.

None of us is right all the time but the price of inaction is just too high. Some good advice here is to trust your gut instincts and to use that indefinable midwife's intuition! If this chapter has not yet convinced you that safeguarding children is all important, then I must urge you to read Victoria Climbié's compelling story. Safeguarding children is difficult, emotionally highly charged and extremely time-consuming, but it is worthwhile. If you prevent just one child from experiencing harm during your career you will have done a great job.

🔑 Key points

- Safeguarding children is everybody's concern and responsibility.
- Existing legislation and related government information offer a framework to inform practice – make sure that you are familiar with national and local guidance.
- Timely referral, inter-agency collaboration and effective information sharing are fundamental to underpinning good practice.
- Good documentation is crucial – be factual and concise.
- Safeguarding children is a heavy responsibility – access help and support to share the emotional labour.

References

Department for Education and Skills (2006a) *Working Together to Safeguard Children: A Guide to Inter-agency Working to Safeguard and Promote the Welfare of Children*. The Stationery Office, London.

Department for Education and Skills (2006b) *Sharing Information: Practitioners' Guide*. The Stationery Office, London.

Department for Education and Skills (2006c) *The Common Assessment Framework for Children and Young People: Practitioners' Guide*. The Stationery Office, London.

Department for Education and Skills (2006d) *What To Do If You Are Worried a Child is Being Abused*. The Stationery Office, London.

DH (2002) *Learning from Past Experience – A Review of Serious Case Reviews*. The Stationery Office, London.

DH (2003) Every child matters. *Green Paper: Working Together to Safeguard Children*. The Stationery Office, London.

DH (2004) *The NSF for Children, Young People and Maternity Services*. The Stationery Office, London.

Dyer, C. (1993) Families sue over children harmed in hospital. *British Medical Journal*, **306** (6883), 952–954.

Great Britain (1989) *The Children Act 1989 (c41)*, HMSO, London.

Great Britain (1990) *Human Fertilization and Embryology Act 1990 (c37)*, HMSO, London.

Great Britain (1998) *Human Rights Act 1998 (c42)*, HMSO, London.

Great Britain (2003a) *Sexual Offences Act 2003 (c42)*, HMSO, London.

Great Britain (2003b) *Female Genital Mutilation Act 2003 (c31)*, HMSO, London.

Great Britain (2004a) *Domestic Violence Crime and Victims Act 2004 (c28)*, HMSO, London.

Great Britain (2004b) *The Children Act 2004 (c31)*, HMSO, London.

Lee, B. (2007) FGM: an outmoded practice? *Midwives*. Royal College of Midwives, London.

Lord Laming (2003) *The Victoria Climbié Inquiry*. HMSO, Norwich.

McMahon, N. (2005) I blame the parents. *Inform*. Reynolds Porter Chamberlain, London.

NMC (2004a) *The NMC Code of Professional Conduct, Standards for Conduct, Performance and Ethics*. Nursing and Midwifery Council, London.

NMC (2004b) *Midwives Rules and Standards*. Nursing and Midwifery Council, London.

Pearsall, J. and Trumble, W. (eds) (2002) *Oxford English Reference Dictionary*. Oxford University Press, Oxford.

Turner, W. (1902) The general medical council special session. *Lancet*, **1** (4096), 626–633.

Complex needs

Perinatal mental health

Sarah Snow

'Nothing could have prepared me for the realisation that I was a mother, one of the givens, when I knew I was in a state of creation myself.' Rich, quoted in Suleiman (1985: 356)

Twenty-first century midwifery care is informed by a variety of key public health issues, including perinatal mental health. The care of women with perinatal mental health problems occupies a fragile space within contemporary healthcare environments. The rise of evidence-based medicine, with the Cochrane Collaboration at its core, is coupled closely with the government's public health agenda, and overburdened community midwives are currently presented with complex challenges on a daily basis. This chapter will not centre on the appropriateness of this public health agenda, but it will address the practicalities of such an agenda within the current framework supporting most maternity service provision. The key aim is to demonstrate that women's mental health demands more attention.

In order to develop the aim of this chapter further, it is necessary to first explain what it is not. I have no specific clinical expertise in mental health nursing. Instead, my knowledge and understanding are drawn from midwifery experiences of supporting women in the community, and being witness to their complex transition along the unknown road to motherhood. This chapter does not claim to be a definitive guide to the broad range of emotional and psychiatric disturbances that can affect women at any stage during the childbearing process, but it will explore perinatal mental health issues from the perspectives of women and of midwives who are perhaps new to the community setting. After reading, and hopefully enjoying, this chapter the reader will be able to:

- refresh their knowledge about the mild and moderate mood disorders that affect women following childbirth
- understand the key differences between these disorders and puerperal psychosis
- consider a range of midwifery strategies for supporting women with compromised mental health states, both urgent and planned
- obtain an introduction to post-traumatic stress disorder and tokophobia
- identify and locate current evidence and additional resources
- locate perinatal mental health within a broader sociological and feminist context
- explore personal beliefs surrounding mental health and consequential impact on women's care.

Historical perspective

Women's temporary 'madness' around the time of childbearing has been recognised since the time of Hippocrates (cited in Cox, 1986), with Marce being the first physician to accurately describe the pathological effects of anxiety during pregnancy in the 18th century. Medicine's response to women's altered mental health states has varied through the ages, frequently influenced by current practices and cultural norms, and often within patriarchal assumptions about women's bodies and 'normal' responses to motherhood. Plato is commonly held responsible for proposing the belief that the root of women's emotional disturbance could be located within the 'wandering womb' theory, meaning essentially that a woman's mental health could only be stable when her womb was used 'properly' or 'naturally' for childbearing. However, Dixon (1995) contends that this perception may well have arisen from beliefs held by the ancient Egyptians that were subsequently adopted by Greek scholars. As a consequence, women have been viewed throughout history as being at the mercy of their fluctuating reproductive cycles: out of control and unable to function 'normally' within the public sphere enjoyed and dominated by men (Oakley, 1993). This perspective of women's health has persisted through time, echoes of which can be seen in gynaecological language that reinforces the incompetence of women's bodies and minds: 'blighted ovum', 'melancholia', 'incompetent cervix'. There is some evidence, however, that attitudes are changing. The Royal College of Obstetricians and Gynaecologists (RCOG, 2006) recently published guidelines relating to the management of early pregnancy loss, recommending that terms such as 'blighted ovum' be abandoned because of the emotional distress they are likely to cause women and their families.

The medical beliefs historically related to the origins of women's mental illness can be challenged in a number of ways, but some aspects of the treatment offered may actually have helped women. In parts of Victorian England, for example, women who experienced non-psychotic mental health problems following childbirth were admitted to pauper asylums. Here they were allowed to rest over a period of several months whilst engaging in simple tasks that were deemed to be therapeutic. The story of Sarah Drabble offers some insight (Box 9.1).

Box 9.1 Sarah Drabble's story

Sarah Drabble, aged 37, was admitted to the West Riding pauper asylum on 15 September 1832 'in a low desponding state'. She had 18 children and her thyroid gland was noted to be enlarged. Following a period of treatment that included the application of leeches, the ingestion of various oils and potions, boosting appetite and rest, Sarah was 'discharged cured' on 25 December 1832.

History to Herstory Archive (2007)

Although the concept of a woman being compulsorily admitted to an asylum is disturbing, the companionship and simple measures on offer within their walls share similarities with contemporary strategies for the support of postnatal women experiencing emotional distress in the 21st century.

There are a range of terms relating to perinatal mental health that may be unfamiliar to midwives who have had limited exposure to concepts of mental health during their midwifery training. As recently as the 1980s, there was very little in the course content beyond the brief inclusion of the topic of puerperal psychosis. There was certainly nothing about the wider context of women's lives influencing mental health and related feminist theory. Ironically, the psychiatric placements in general nurse training exposed many pre-registered midwifery students during the late 20th century to women who had been confined to institutions for many years with original, yet vague, diagnoses of postnatal illness.

It is appropriate, at this point, to clarify some of the associated terminology to refresh the reader's knowledge and also because this is of critical importance for midwives working in the community setting.

Postnatal 'blues'

This transient episode is familiar to midwives as the 'baby' or 'third day' blues. It is characterised by fluctuating moods of general weepiness and euphoria, and occurs frequently to affect 30–75% of women (Seyfried and Marcus, 2003). It requires only time and support to resolve. Anecdote and experience suggest that the majority of mid-wives anticipate that nearly all women will experience an episode of the 'blues'. Many midwives believe the cause to be the result of massive changes in circulating pregnancy hormones, although this is not established. Henshaw (2003) suggests that the only credible evidence is a link between the 'blues' and dysphoria during pregnancy. Dysphoria has been described as a state of feeling unwell, or unhappy (Medline Plus, 2007).

This is an important link because it highlights that women can experience depression and unhappiness during the antenatal as well as postnatal periods. Antenatal depression receives much less attention, although prevalence rates are believed to be substantial (Bennett et al., 2004).

Brockington (1996) identifies that there are conflicting findings relating to the neurochemical changes and development of the 'blues'. Some studies show a correlation with progesterone and others do not. Brockington's analysis of the evidence suggests that the role of catecholamines in the development of the 'blues' is the only theory to emerge with a degree of validity. It was demonstrated almost 40 years ago by research that found reduced levels of urinary noradrenaline in women 3 days after birth (Treadway et al., 1969; cited in Brockington, 1996) (Box 9.2). Noradrenaline is a neurotransmitter, known to influence a range of physiological and psychological processes. Disorders of this neurotransmitter system are implicated in a range of psychiatric disturbances (Brunello et al., 2003). Although women recover from an episode of the 'blues' and it is generally perceived to be a fleeting mood change (Brockington, 1996), it is important to remember that the 'blues' has a moderate to strong association with the development of postnatal depression (Beck, 1996; O'Hara and Swain, 1996; Wilson et al., 1996).

Box 9.2 Summary of third day 'blues'

- Characterised by dysphoric mood.
- Transient.
- Possibly related to catecholamine levels.
- Postnatal depression can develop from prolonged 'blues'.

Postnatal depression

This is a much more complex condition on several fronts. There are numerous and competing definitions, aetiologies and prevalence rates. Community midwives may have limited exposure to women suffering from postnatal depression because it may not occur until several weeks following birth, but evidence has shown that women do experience episodes of depression within 4 weeks of birth (Cox et al., 1993).

Feminists question the labelling of postnatal depression as an illness, instead suggesting that women experience depressive symptoms as a normal response to motherhood, especially within a patriarchal society (Nicolson, 1993; Oakley, 1993). However, there is no doubt that depression is a common condition. It affects a large number of women and is responsible for a great deal of distress and unhappiness. Prevalence rates for postnatal depression are 10–15% of women (Seyfried and Marcus, 2003). Oakley (1993) has commented that it should be no surprise that many women experience postnatal depression. Her sociological viewpoint leans towards an anticipation that all women are at risk of this disabling disorder.

The World Health Organization predicts that depression will be the second greatest cause of premature mortality and morbidity worldwide by 2020 (Murray and Lopez, 1996). Given that the leading cause overall of maternal death is psychiatric illness (Lewis, 2004), evidence to support this prediction is already available (Box 9.3).

Box 9.3 Practice point

In terms of psychiatric illness and maternal death, there is a critical window of 3 months before and 3 months after birth when women are especially vulnerable.

Lewis (2004)

Competing perspectives relating to postnatal depression warrant exploration, both to clarify the debate and demonstrate to the reader that a broader and deeper focus is required if the mental health needs of women, and consequently their families, are to be met. It is also timely to reiterate that a significant proportion of women experience depression in the antenatal period (Evans et al., 2001).

Medical model

The medical model of postnatal depression concentrates on the complex interface of hormonal and endocrine processes during childbearing (Gregoire, 1995). Dalton (1980) put forward the theory some time ago that the sudden fall in progesterone levels following birth were responsible for postnatal depression and recommended the use of progesterone supplements. Her studies were uncontrolled and their methodological rigor has been brought into question. In contrast, Meakin and Brockington (1990) found that progesterone was ineffective in the treatment of puerperal mania and Gregoire (1995) suggested that prolonged exposure to progesterone could actually exacerbate depressive symptoms. A review by Karuppaswamy and Vlies (2003) reinforced this by highlighting that synthetic progesterone is associated with depression in the postnatal period, although it might still be used with caution in some cases. Overall, there does not appear to be any evidence for the use of natural or synthetic progestogens in the treatment of postnatal depression (Lawrie et al., 2001).

Gregoire (1995) suggests that thyroid hormones have a clear and established link with depressive illness. This is based on physiological evidence that a disturbance of thyroid function can affect mood and produce symptoms of anxiety. Secondly, where the thyroid hormone tri-iodothyronine is used in combination with antidepressant drugs the overall therapeutic effect is augmented and enhanced (Lifschytz et al., 2006). Harris (1993) estimated that 10% of women with postnatal depression have thyroid function disturbance and found that 6–7% of women in their study suffered from abnormal, but usually self-limiting, thyroid function in the postpartum period. Cooper and Murray (1998) contest this data as unsubstantiated and suggest that the thyroid dysfunction could be secondary to immunological changes caused by stress. More recent clinical trials (Harris et al., 2002) found thyroxine to be ineffective in the treatment of postnatally depressed women who had abnormal thyroid function.

Current best evidence suggests that risk factors for postnatal depression are no different to the risk factors for any other depressive illness (SIGN, 2002). For community midwives working with women in a variety of social and economic circumstances, it is important to note that the strongest associations with postnatal depression are, amongst others, a low level of social support, poor marital relationship and recent life events (Beck, 1996; O'Hara and Swain, 1996; Wilson et al., 1996). Evidence relating to specific factors such as obstetric complications is much weaker but this does not rule them out altogether, especially when they appear to be significant in the aetiology of emerging mental health problems such as tokophobia.

The sociological context associated with the development of postnatal depression will be explored next. This essentially forms the basis of a feminist approach that can underpin an understanding of women's unhappiness following childbirth.

Sociological context

Becoming a mother requires a woman to undergo a fundamental transition to assume a new and complex identity (Richardson, 1993). Feminist debate focuses on the concept of dissonance, or tension, between the expectations of this new identity and the realities of motherhood. This dissonance is further compounded by the perception embedded within patriarchy that motherhood is a 'natural' and inevitable state that all women naturally aspire to (Richardson, 1993; Smart, 1996). The stark realities of staying at home to care for young children were first described from a critical perspective by Oakley (1979). In her qualitative study, women articulated the relentless demands placed upon them, the frequently mundane tasks of childcare and the low value placed upon this unpaid work. Above all, these women described their loneliness.

In the Western world, women largely mother their children in isolation, away from traditional sources of support and companionship found in an extended family and network of friends (Rokach, 2004). This is partly due to demographic and economic changes that have seen a dispersal of extended families across the UK and a diminishing birth rate (Office for National Statistics, 2005). Women therefore have little opportunity to witness other members of their family engaged in mothering tasks such as breastfeeding. Consequently, they have limited access to positive role models. The inherent loneliness of the mothering experience therefore contradicts the appealing 'wholesome' image of motherhood that is entwined with femininity and perpetuated within a patriarchal society (Box 9.4).

Box 9.4 What is patriarchy?

Patriarchy is a feminist theory (there are many other feminist theories) that suggests male dominance over all the significant elements of societal function. It confines women and renders them subordinate.

Traditionally, men have controlled the public spheres of religion, state, medicine and law, and actively sought to confine women to the private sphere of home and domesticity.

Currently, more women than men enter medical school, but only 22% of women have attained the position of consultant within the field of general medicine (Royal College of Physicians, 2004).

There is also a continued controversy regarding the ordination of women priests and women account for only 34% of judicial posts (Judicial Studies Board, 2002).

Adcock (1993) suggests that the conflict between a woman's expectations and the reality of her experiences as a new mother, combined with the struggle to meet the expectations of society, can explain the development of postnatal depression. This conflict is in addition to the numerous and enormous life changes that a new mother has to negotiate, frequently in isolation and without support. This critical adaptation has been described within the context of a grieving model (Nicolson, 1998), where there is conflict between the 'special' status of new motherhood and acute feelings of loss for independence, lifestyle and camaraderie. Additionally, there is the experience of a displaced position in society. Where a woman has succeeded in gaining some recognition within the public world of her working life, she then has to retreat to the private world of domesticity where this work is considered to have little value. This dissonance is further compounded by the inherent contradictions of mothering that range from deep desperation to moments of sheer joy. This is classically described by Rich (1984: 21) as 'the suffering of ambivalence'.

This feminist perspective can, of course, be challenged. Firstly, there is the assumption that all women find motherhood oppressive, yet becoming a mother can be a deeply satisfying and uplifting experience. It can also be the source of a paradox that leads to a degree of confusion and guilt (Parker, 1995). A prime example relates to the woman who is compelled to return to work. Delegating the care of your baby to others is an unacknowledged and emotionally overwhelming experience for many women. Richardson (1993) suggests that it is not motherhood that oppresses women but the conditions in which women are expected to mother. Working mothers with children under the age of 5 now make up half of the labour force in the UK (Office of National Statistics, 2004) and continue to struggle with a sustained lack of affordable, good quality childcare provision. One aim of the current evaluation of the Sure Start project is to illuminate the effectiveness of supporting working mothers and their children in areas of social deprivation, and to highlight the potential benefits to their mutual health (Birkbeck College, University of London, 2007).

Secondly, the experience of motherhood has been dominated by the experiences of white women, thereby assuming that all women are the same. There is evidence to suggest that women from minority ethnic groups prize family life as a vital shield against racism (Jackson, 1993).

How then, does this complex and controversial debate apply to a community midwife going about her daily business? Well, it is no longer possible for midwives to separate themselves from the political and social constructs that affect women's lives. Inadequate social support as a cause of depression is frequently secondary to other significant problems affecting mental health, such as poverty (Seguin, 1999). There may be limited value in providing supportive social networks where fundamental inequalities remain ignored and unaddressed. As midwives, we cannot solve fundamental health inequalities in isolation, but we are in a position to agitate for alternative patterns of maternity care that maximise women's childbirth and parenting choices, when choices may be limited elsewhere in their lives.

Midwifery care of women with depression

We have seen that the aetiology of postnatal depression is both complex and controversial. Incidences and timings vary and this means that it is impossible to put postnatal depression into a convenient diagnostic box. Brockington (1996) is sceptical regarding narrow concepts of postnatal depression, and the need for emotional distress to be seen in a much broader context is echoed elsewhere (White et al., 2006). Brockington (1996) states that this issue should assume greater importance because it legitimises maternal depression and highlights the fact that depression following birth is clinically similar to depression occurring at any other time in a woman's life.

Women may be sad, anxious, irritable and tense. In a mild form, these symptoms will be recognised as being common amongst the roller-coaster of emotions that women can experience in the early days of motherhood. Community midwives must therefore be alert to the significance of such symptoms for the woman, especially if they are prolonged. But the challenge lies in distinguishing the features relating to what is an essentially normal reaction to motherhood from depressive symptoms suggestive of illness. Health visitors have traditionally used specific screening tools to assist them with this task; the most commonly used is the Edinburgh Postnatal Depression Scale (EPDS). Although there are many criticisms of the EPDS, for example its questionable transferability to women from minority ethnic groups, SIGN (2002) and NICE (2007) advise that the EPDS should continue to be offered to women as part of a screening programme at approximately 6 weeks and 3 months following birth.

To help focus the reader's thinking, it is always useful to introduce a case study. The story of 'Louise' is one that I use when discussing postnatal depression in the classroom with senior student midwives and it always provokes a lot of discussion (Case study 9.1). Many of these students have never had the opportunity to support women beyond 10 days after a birth, despite the fact that the need for extended support is often very obvious.

Case study 9.1 The story of 'Louise'

You are a community midwife who has been caring for Louise since her discharge from hospital: you are visiting again today, 3 weeks after the birth of her first baby, Chloe.

Louise had a ventouse delivery for delay in the second stage of labour and has struggled with breastfeeding. You are still visiting to provide breastfeeding support. Louise's physical recovery has largely been uneventful, apart from an episiotomy that is not completely healed and she is taking iron supplements for an Hb of 9.6.

You enjoy a good relationship with Louise and have known her professionally since 28 weeks' gestation. She is also the teacher of your own children at the local primary school.

During the visit, Chloe is asleep in her pram. Louise looks pale and tired. You sense that she is close to tears and sure enough, as you gently enquire how she feels, Louise begins to cry. She tells you that she feels very low, is not sleeping and doesn't feel able to cope anymore.

You may have identified the following points for discussion:

- extended postnatal support visits
- integrated care pathways
- demands of breastfeeding and sources of support
- expectations/realities of new motherhood
- postnatal sadness or postnatal depression?
- midwife as friend
- referral to others and treatment options, e.g. anti-depressants/counselling
- other sources of support, e.g. consumer groups
- interprofessional networking
- promotion of wound healing.

Whatever midwives may think about Louise's diagnosis, the reality for her at this current time is one of compromised mental health. Macrory (2005) highlights the simple fact that there is no health without mental health. If we view compromised mental health as being no different to compromised physical health, then we have a duty to respond to Louise's health needs. With mild mood disorders, this response can be surprisingly little. The National Association for Mental Health (MIND, 2006) found that women want the support of healthcare professionals who are able to foster a trusting relationship based on understanding and sensitivity. Community midwives, who enjoy the privilege of really 'knowing' women and their families, are ideally placed to provide this support and to foster a professional friendship with the women in their care. Women want to have a special relationship with midwives, and do not expect the same relationship with other health professionals (Pairman, 2000). Student midwives appear to be especially skilled at forming meaningful relationships with women because they share the experience of 'newness' and relative powerlessness (Snow, 2006). However, the question of professional boundaries and accountability does not sit comfortably with this perspective, and further work is needed to specifically define what women expect from their 'friendship' with midwives. For example, what is the inherent nature of the knowledge, skills, attitudes and behaviour of midwives that women locate their perceptions of friendship within? As Pairman (2000) suggests, the concept of partnership with women is preferable because of the centrality of power sharing within this type of relationship.

Although the provision of specific and targeted support visits by health visitors has not been found to reduce rates of depressive illness, women evaluate the additional support positively (Wiggins et al., 2004). Dennis (2005), in her systematic review of psychosocial interventions for the treatment of postnatal depression, suggests that the additional support measures provided by professionals in the postnatal period remain the most promising intervention in the prevention of depression. She concludes that further research is required in order to substantiate this intervention further and a broader perspective of women's experiences is particularly desirable. Although we need to explore this type of intervention more fully, NICE (2007) highlights listening visits as a key strategy in the support of depressed women.

As student midwives point out when discussing 'Louise's' care, women are frequently discharged to the care of health visitors at the statutory minimum of 10 days. Health visitors then have responsibility for the monitoring and support of women's mental health. There are examples of integrated care pathways that support health visitors in this vital role but they are not universally accessible at present.

The organisation of most maternity care systems and problems with the retention of practising midwives significantly limits midwifery opportunities to support women with depression occurring a few weeks after birth (Box 9.5). This represents a lost opportunity, both in the context of therapeutic relationships with women that may have been established over some time, and the development of specific skills that assist midwives in the support of women experiencing unhappiness following birth.

Box 9.5 Summary: postnatal depression

- Not clearly defined.
- Long-term morbidity effects on woman and her family.
- Postnatal depression should be viewed within a broader context.
- Evidence supporting varied treatment strategies is not robust – targeted support by healthcare professionals appears most promising.

Puerperal psychosis

There are many severe psychiatric disorders that can affect women around the time of childbirth, and their scope and complexity are outside the remit of this chapter. One condition familiar to midwives, and specific to childbearing women, is puerperal psychosis. This is a relatively rare, serious illness that affects approximately 1–2 women per 1000 and typically presents within the first postpartum month (SIGN, 2002). Risk factors for the development of psychosis are distinctly different from postnatal illness (Table 9.1). Note that community midwives are generally more likely to see puerperal psychosis than postnatal depression.

Unlike the mild depressive symptoms that many women experience in the antenatal and postnatal periods, the symptoms of puerperal psychosis are severe and reflect those of other psychiatric psychotic

Table 9.1 Risk factors for postnatal illness and puerperal psychosis.

Postnatal illness	Puerperal psychosis
• Past history • Low social support • Poor marital relationship • Recent life events • 'Baby blues' O'Hara and Swain (1996) Beck (1996) Wilson et al. (1996)	Past history • Pre-existing and severe psychotic illness • Family history in first/second degree relatives McNeil (1987) Benvenuti et al (1992) Marks et al (1992) Schopf and Rust (1994)

illness. Broadly, these include hallucinations, abnormal behaviour, lack of insight and severe thought disturbance (SIGN, 2002). Oates (2005) memorably recounted the behaviour of one woman, admitted to a psychiatric unit and experiencing puerperal psychosis, who ran freely around the ward entirely naked. Although this story gently amused her conference audience, the distress experienced by the woman's family was equally highlighted – the rapid onset of bizarre and uncharacteristic behaviour can be extremely frightening to all concerned and the sequelae potentially catastrophic. In the last CEMD report (Lewis, 2004), 28 women had killed themselves, and sometimes their infant and older children too, because of severe psychiatric illness that was frequently not recognised or appropriately managed.

Less spectacular symptoms of developing psychosis can also include behaviour that is generally confused or vague. These symptoms can be much more difficult for a community midwife to assess accurately, especially if she has not met the woman before (Box 9.6).

Box 9.6 Practice point: puerperal psychosis

- Regular updates within community teams need to revisit the signs and symptoms of puerperal psychosis, particularly where a woman displays less marked features of developing illness.
- Help and support must be accessed promptly.
- As a minimum, there should be clear referral pathways to specialist emergency psychiatric support teams, or access to an on-call consultant psychiatrist/mother and baby unit.

For some time now, I have held the belief that puerperal psychosis should be viewed in the same way as any other acute obstetric emergency. Community midwives should initiate an appropriate sequence of events in response to psychotic illness, just as they would in response to shoulder dystocia or cord prolapse at a home birth.

Puerperal psychosis responds well to appropriate treatment and women generally make a full recovery, although they are at significant risk of further perinatal and other psychotic illness (McNeil, 1987; Benvenuti et al., 1992; Robling et al., 2000). Specialist units that provide care and treatment for women suffering with puerperal psychosis, whilst their babies remain with them, are a precious commodity in the UK, where there are just eight units in total. This means that many women will be treated on general psychiatric wards where their specific needs as new mothers may not be fully met. Women prize the care and treatment offered within mother and baby units, often initiating local campaigns to agitate for more services (Flanagan, 2007), although Joy and Saylan (2007) suggest that the clinical and economic value of such services has not yet been robustly evaluated.

The CEMD (Lewis, 2004) has once more found that psychiatric illness is the leading cause of maternal death overall. Of the women who died, 28 committed suicide, all by violent means and some along-side their babies and other children. Most of these women had known histories of previous psychiatric illness, yet most did not have a plan of care. As with most cases of maternal death, communication failure is often the most significant contributory factor to poor care. Although there are clear cases within the CEMD report of women taking their own lives despite excellent communication and inter-professional working, many of these catastrophic deaths should have been avoided (Box 9.7).

Box 9.7 Practice point: information sharing

The *Confidential Enquiries into Maternal Deaths* (Lewis, 2004) found that *all* of the relevant information relating to *all* of the women's previous and/or current illness could be found in GP records. Until the age of electronic patient held records, community midwives are advised to exploit this information more fully.

One of the recommendations from the CEMD report (Lewis, 2004) focuses on the critical importance of avoiding the generic term 'post-natal illness' on antenatal booking notes. Not only does this term have many interpretations, as we have seen in this chapter, it may also disguise a more serious psychiatric history and delay or prevent a woman from receiving appropriate care. Many maternity units now incorporate integrated care pathways to ensure that significant information is shared, thus minimising the mortality risks associated with serious psychotic illness.

Post-traumatic stress disorder

Post-traumatic stress disorder (PTSD) is not a new phenomenon. It was first seen, although not always given appropriate recognition, during the World War I. Traumatised and damaged young men returning from trench warfare were described as being 'shell-shocked'. In her review, Andreasen (2004: 1321) explains that PTSD only emerged as a medical diagnosis following World War II, where soldiers were again exposed to significant stressors that were 'outside the range of normal human experience'.

In the modern world, people are at risk of developing PTSD if they are exposed to major stressors such as rape, abuse or terrorism. Beck (2004) contends that childbirth is a potent stressor and cites the range of women who experience PTSD as 1.5–6%. However, exposure to a major stressful event does not automatically equate with the development of PTSD. Ayers (2003) comments that there are important distinctions between the perception of traumatic birth, a stress response and clinical PTSD: although inter-related, these three concepts are still distinct. Women may display symptoms of a stress response to their birth experience yet recover normally without the development of significant clinical features. Although the evidence base relating to PTSD and childbirth is currently patchy with further research required, several risk factors have been suggested. It is important to note that there is no consistent evidence to support these risk factors (Ayers, 2003) and this has important implications for midwives who participate in postnatal debriefing (Box 9.8).

Box 9.8 Labour/birth risk factors for post-traumatic stress disorder

- Emergency LSCS (Ryding et al., 1997).
- Instrumentally assisted births (MacLean et al., 2000).
- Memories of past sexual abuse can be triggered by certain events in labour and cause re-traumatisation (Crompton, 1996).
- Signs of possible re-traumatisation in women (where events trigger memories of previous trauma) during labour can include withdrawal, loss of control and severe distress.

Perceptions of control and cognitive factors

Lyons (1998) and Czarnocka and Slade (2000) found that women were less likely to develop PTSD where they felt in control during their labour and knew what to expect. The issue of women's perceptions of control is a major theme that consistently emerges in the literature exploring women's experiences of childbirth (Gibbins and Thompson, 2001). What is perhaps more complex is the disparity between women's and midwives' perceptions of control (Case study 9.2).

Case study 9.2 Midwife's perception of control

Women in antenatal support groups have often shared stories of their previous births with me to demonstrate the conflict between consumer and carer perceptions. For example, one midwife's documentation indicated that a woman's labour progressed rapidly and without any complications to culminate in a 'normal' spontaneous birth. Yet the woman felt traumatised by the rapid sequence of events and delayed a second pregnancy as a result.

Some evidence suggests that trait anxiety and dysfunctional attitudes may increase the risk of PTSD, although further research is needed (Czarnocka and Slade, 2000; Grazioli and Terry, 2000). Trait anxiety refers to individual differences in proneness to anxiety. It is the general term given to individuals who usually respond with anxiety to perceived threats in their environment (Spielberger, 1983) (Case study 9.3).

Case study 9.3 Trait anxiety

A woman who had experienced an emergency hysterectomy after a primary postpartum haemorrhage needed gynaecological follow up. It took several attempts over a number of weeks before she was able to attend her appointment. The approach to the hospital triggered acutely distressing memories of her experience that manifested in panic attacks.

The consequences of traumatic childbirth that results in PTSD are complex, prolonged, severely debilitating and will affect the family unit (Ayers et al., 2006). Women can suffer flashbacks, nightmares and acute anxiety long after the original stressor.

De-briefing services

In an effort to combat the development of PTSD and to support women with other forms of postpartum emotional distress, midwives are becoming increasingly involved with de-briefing services. These offer an opportunity for women to discuss their care and to ask questions, rather than providing a counselling service. Bailham and Joseph (2003) suggest that this type of de-briefing is potentially helpful and enables referral to specialist services where appropriate. Ayers et al. (2006), however, are much more cautious. They suggest that the outcomes of postnatal de-briefing have produced conflicting results and are not necessarily targeted at women experiencing PTSD. They further question the limited scope of midwifery-led de-briefing as opposed to structured psychological interventions. As with all other aspects of perinatal mental health, much more research is needed in order to support midwives who currently engage with postnatal de-briefing to ensure that women receive an effective, therapeutic service. This is particularly important for severely distressed, vulnerable women and, at present, NICE (2005) does not recommend de-briefing for any adult experiencing PTSD.

Tokophobia

Tokophobia, or an 'unreasoning dread of childbirth', is a relatively new phenomenon in the medical literature, although the care of women who refuse the experience of vaginal birth will not be unfamiliar to many community midwives. Whether this refusal is because of 'unreasoning dread', and therefore linked with compromised mental health, or because of 'normal' anxiety relating to fear of the unknown, is open to debate. Walsh (2002) suggests that tokophobia is a consequence of medicalised birth. However, we must consider this fear and anxiety as a problem regardless because it clearly impacts on women's experiences of childbirth and hence their midwifery care. In particular, tokophobia is clearly linked to PTSD. Ayers et al. (2006) explored the effects of childbirth-related PTSD on women's health, and identified fear of subsequent childbirth as one serious and lasting consequence.

Hofberg and Brockington (2000) currently lead a very small field in the exploration of the concept of tokophobia. In one small study, they found that 13% of women either postponed or avoided pregnancy completely because of their extreme fear and anxiety. From their analysis and subsequent work, Hofberg and Ward (2003) offer a further classification of the illness as primary and secondary tokophobia. The relevant causal factors identified in their research are listed for clarity in Table 9.2.

Table 9.2 Classification for tokophobia.

Primary – nulliparous	Secondary – to previous traumatic birth	Secondary – to depressive illness
• Social influence, e.g. transmission of fear through generations • Trauma/abuse • Anxiety theories	• Linked to PTSD • Emergency LSCS • Instrumental delivery • Expectations/ experiences	• Uncommon • Can present with antenatal depression

It is unsurprising that factors such as sexual trauma are a primary cause of tokophobia. The experience of childbirth can frequently render women powerless. Both the physical sensations during birth and the practices employed by midwives can serve to painfully remind women of their abuse (Barlow and Birch, 2004). For many of these women, vaginal birth is simply not an option.

At a different level, there is a valid concern that societal and cultural influences over generations may have unwittingly provoked extreme fear of childbirth. Major shifts in the social meaning of childbirth over the past century are well documented (Donnison, 1988). Women have always shared birth stories amongst each other as a part of childbirth ritual and tradition, yet fewer women today have an opportunity to witness the process of childbirth directly. As a result, they have no point of reference that enables them to put other women's stories into an appropriate context.

Women have always supported each other during birth by encouraging, distracting and attending to the emotional and physical needs of the labouring woman. This shared support maximised the normality of birth and kept it firmly within the realms of women's business. Subsequent medicalisation of birth has refocused this perspective to one where birth is no longer viewed within its broader social context but rather as something to be managed, feared and controlled. With high rates of operative deliveries further reducing women's experience of normal birth, it could be seen as a forgone conclusion that real fear has become embedded into some women's perceptions of the nature of childbirth. This consequence of medicalisation, and indeed others, has been described as disastrous to the future health and happiness of women in particular and society in general (Wagner, 2002).

More optimistically, there is some evidence to suggest that it is possible to help women manage anxiety and reduce fear of childbirth. Saisto et al. (2001) found that a structured programme of interventions by trained obstetricians and midwives enabled women to address anxiety and make birth choices that otherwise would have been closed to them. Although this could be seen as merely undoing the damage inherent within medicalised birth, it nevertheless serves to remind midwives that the essence of women's needs are not difficult to meet, provided that adequate time and support are available.

Summary

It is hoped that this chapter has provided the reader with an overview of some of the conditions and issues that affect women's perinatal mental health. It did not set out to provide an in-depth exploration of particular aspects. For instance, the ranges of pharmacological treatments for the management of depression have not been examined, but signposts to further relevant material have been included. Overall, this chapter has aimed to equip midwives who are new to a role in the community with additional material that will be helpful in developing therapeutic relationships with women. The key message contained within that material is quite straightforward: women's perinatal mental health needs demand far greater attention, not least because the failure to do so can have catastrophic consequences. Perinatal mental health must also be contextualised within the experience of becoming a mother because the reality of that experience has a direct, and sometimes prolonged, impact on women's emotional health.

Key points

- Community midwives must maximise their partnership with women in order to recognise and support normal emotional reactions to motherhood.
- Antenatal depression is at least as common as postnatal depression.
- All community midwives must be familiar with referral pathways for women who become seriously distressed in the antenatal or postnatal periods.
- The generic term 'postnatal depression' must be used with caution.
- The consequences of maternal depression can be prolonged, severe and extend to impact significantly upon a woman's children and family.
- Further research is urgently needed to explore support systems in the context of depression prevention and women's experiences of contemporary motherhood.

References

Adcock, J. (1993) Expectations they cannot meet. *Professional Nurse*, 8, 703–710.

Andreasen, N. (2004) Acute and delayed post-traumatic stress disorders: a history and some issues. *American Journal of Psychiatry*, **161** (8), 1321–1323.

Ayers, S. (2003) Commentary on 'post-traumatic stress following childbirth: a review of the emerging literature and directions for research and practice'. *Psychology, Health and Medicine*, **8** (2), 169–171.

Ayers, S., Eagle, A. and Waring, H. (2006) The effects of childbirth-related post-traumatic stress disorder on women and their relationships: a qualitative study. *Psychology, Health and Medicine*, **11** (4), 389–398.

Bailham, D. and Joseph, S. (2003) Post-traumatic stress following childbirth: a review of the emerging literature and directions for research and practice. *Psychology, Health and Medicine*, **8** (2), 159–168.

Barlow, J. and Birch, L. (2004) Midwifery practice and sexual abuse. *British Journal of Midwifery*, **12** (2), 72–75.

Beck, C. (1996) A meta-analysis of predictors of postpartum depression. *Nursing Research*, **45**, 297–303.

Beck, C. (2004) Post-traumatic stress disorder due to childbirth: the aftermath. *Nursing Research*, **53** (4), 216–224.

Bennett, H., Einarson, A., Taddio, A., Koren, G. and Einarson, T. (2004) Prevalence of depression during pregnancy: systematic review. *Obstetrics & Gynecology*, **103**, 698–709.

Benvenuti, P., Cabras, P.L., Servi, P., Rosseti, S., Marchetti, G. and Pazzagli, A. (1992) Puerperal psychoses: a clinical case study with follow-up. *Journal of Affective Disorders*, **26**, 25–30.

Birkbeck College, University of London. *National Evaluation of Sure Start*. Institute for the Study of Children, Families & Social Issues. http://www.ness.bbk.ac.uk/ (accessed May 2007).

Brockington, I. (1996) *Motherhood and Mental Health*. Oxford University Press, UK.

Brunello, N., Blier, P., Judd, L., et al. (2003) Noradrenaline in mood and anxiety disorders: basic and clinical studies. *International Clinical Psychopharmacology*, **18** (4), 191–202.

Cooper, P. and Murray, L. (1998) Postnatal depression. *British Medical Journal*, **3** (16), 1884–1886.

Cox, J.L. (1986) *Postnatal Depression: A Guide for Health Professionals*. Churchill Livingstone, Edinburgh.

Cox, J.L., Murray, D. and Chapman, G. (1993) A controlled study of the onset, duration and prevalence of postnatal depression. *British Journal of Psychiatry*, **163**, 27–31.

Crompton, J. (1996) Post-traumatic stress disorder and childbirth. *British Journal of Midwifery*, **4**, 290–293.

Czarnocka, J. and Slade, P. (2000) Prevalence and predictors of post-traumatic stress symptoms following childbirth. *British Journal of Clinical Psychology*, **39**, 35–51.

Dalton, K. (1980) *Depression after Childbirth*. Oxford University Press, Oxford.

Dennis, C.L. (2005) Psychosocial and psychological interventions for prevention of postnatal depression: systematic review. *British Medical Journal*, **331** (7507), 15–23.

Dixon, L. (1995) *Perilous Chastity: Women and Illness in Pre-Enlightenment Art and Medicine*. Cornell University Press, New York.

Donnison, J. (1988) *Midwives and Medical Men: A History for the Struggle for the Control of Childbirth*. Historical Publications, London.

Evans, J., Heron, J., Francomb, H., Oke, S. and Golding, J. (2001) Cohort study of depressed mood during pregnancy and after childbirth. *British Medical Journal*, **323**, 257–260.

Flanagan, A. (2007) Separated at birth. *The Guardian*, 12 February.

Gibbins, J. and Thomson, A. (2001) Women's expectations and experiences of childbirth. *Midwifery*, **17**, 302–313.

Grazioli, R. and Terry, D. (2000) The role of cognitive vulnerability in the prediction of postpartum symptomatology. *British Journal of Clinical Psychology*, **39**, 329–347.

Gregoire, A. (1995) Hormones and postnatal depression. *British Journal of Midwifery*, **3** (2), 99–104.

Harris, B. (1993) A hormonal component to postnatal depression. *British Journal of Psychiatry*, **163**, 403–405.

Harris, B., Oretti, R., Lazarus, J., et al. (2002) Randomised trial of thyroxine to prevent postnatal depression in thyroid-antibody-positive women. *British Journal of Psychiatry*, **180**, 327–330.

Henshaw, C. (2003) Mood disturbance in the early puerperium: a review. *Archives of Women's Mental Health*, **6** (supplement 2), 33–42.

History to Herstory Archive, Yorkshire Women's Lives Online, 1100 to the Present. West Yorkshire Archive Service. http://www.historytoherstory. org.uk/ (accessed May 2007).

Hofberg, K. and Brockington, I. (2000) Tokophobia: an unreasoning dread of childbirth: A series of 26 cases. *British Journal of Psychiatry*, **176**, 83–85.

Hofberg, K. and Ward, M. (2003) Fear of pregnancy and childbirth. *Postgraduate Medical Journal*, **79**, 505–510.

Jackson, S. (1993) Women and the family. In *Introducing Women's Studies* (eds D. Richardson and V. Robinson). MacMillan, London.

Joy, C. and Saylan, M. (2007) Mother and baby units for schizophrenia. *Cochrane Database of Systematic Reviews 2007*, Issue 1, Oxford Update Software.

Judicial Studies Board (2002) Judicial Appointments Annual Report 2001—2002. http://www.dca.gov.uk/judicial/ja_arep2002/chapter1.html#top (accessed January 2007).

Karuppaswamy, J. and Vlies, R. (2003) The benefit of oestrogens and progestogens in postnatal depression. *Journal of Obstetrics and Gynaecology*, **23** (4), 341–346.

Lawrie, T.A., Herxheimer, A. and Dalton, K. (2001) Oestrogens and progestogens for preventing and treating postnatal depression (Cochrane Review). *The Cochrane Library*, Issue 1, Oxford Update Software.

Lewis, G. (2004) *Why Mothers Die 2000–2002, The Sixth Report of the Confidential Enquiries into Maternal Deaths in the United Kingdom*. RCOG Press, London.

Lifschytz, T., Segman, R., Shalom, G., et al. (2006) Basic mechanisms of augmentation of antidepressant effects with thyroid hormone. *Current Drug Targets*, **7** (2), 203–210.

Lyons, S. (1998) A prospective study of post traumatic stress symptoms one month following childbirth. *Journal of Reproductive and Infant Psychology*, **16**, 91–105.

MacLean, L., McDermott, M. and May, C. (2000) Method of delivery and subjective distress: women's emotional responses to childbirth practices. *Journal of Reproductive and Infant Psychology*, **18**, 153–162.

Macrory, F. (2005) Mental illness or social injustice? *Motherhood and the Mind Conference*, Royal Society of Medicine, 23 June 2005.

Marks, M.N., Wieck, A., Checkley, S.A. and Kumar, R. (1992) Contribution of psychological and social factors to psychotic and non-psychotic relapse after childbirth in women with previous histories of affective disorder. *Journal of Affective Disorders*, **24**, 253–263.

McNeil, T. (1987) A prospective study of postpartum psychoses in a high-risk group: relationship to demographic and psychiatric history characteristics. *Acta Psychiatrica Scandinavica*, **75**, 35–43.

Meakin, C. and Brockington, I. (1990) Failure of progesterone treatment in puerperal mania. *British Journal of Psychiatry*, **156**, 910.

MedlinePlus (US National Library of Medicine). http://www.nlm.nih.gov/medlineplus/mplusdictionary.html (accessed May 2007).

MIND (2006) *Out of the Blue? Motherhood and Depression*. MIND, London.

Murray, C. and Lopez, A. (1996) Evidence-based health policy – lessons from the Global Burden of Disease Study. *Science*, **274**, 740–743.

NICE (2005) *The Management of PTSD in Adults and Children in Primary and Secondary Care*. National Institute for Clinical Excellence, London.

NICE (2007) *Antenatal and Postnatal Mental Health*. National Institute for Clinical Excellence, London.

Nicolson, P. (1993) Motherhood and women's lives. In *Introducing Women's Studies* (eds D Richardson and V. Robinson). MacMillan, London.

Nicolson, P. (1998) *Postnatal Depression: Psychology, Science and the Transition to Motherhood*. Routledge, London.

Oakley, A. (1979) *Becoming a Mother*. Martin Robertson, London.

Oakley, A. (1993) *Essays on Women, Medicine and Health*. University Press, Edinburgh.

Oates, M. (2005) Psychiatric causes of maternal death. *Motherhood and the Mind Conference*, Royal Society of Medicine, 23 June 2005.

Office for National Statistics (2004) *Focus on Gender*. http://www.statistics.gov.uk/CCI/nugget.asp?ID=436 (accessed May 2006).

Office for National Statistics (2005) *Birth Statistics: Review of the Registrar General on Births and Patterns of Family Building in England and Wales, 2004*. HMSO, London.

O'Hara, M. and Swain, A. (1996) Rates and risk of postnatal depression – a meta-analysis. *International Review of Psychiatry*, **8**, 37–54.

Pairman, S. (2000) Women-centred midwifery: partnerships or professional friendships? In *The Midwife–Mother Relationship* (ed M. Kirkham). Palgrave MacMillan, Basingstoke.

Parker, R. (1995) *Torn in Two: The Experience of Maternal Ambivalence*. Virago, London.

RCOG (2006) *The Management of Early Pregnancy Loss. Green Top Guideline No 25*. Royal College of Obstetricians and Gynaecologists, London.

Rich, A. (1984) Compulsory heterosexuality and lesbian existence. In *Desire: The Politics of Sexuality* (eds A. Snitow, C. Stansell and S. Thompson). Virago, London.

Richardson, D. (1993) *Women, Motherhood and Childrearing*. MacMillan, London.

Robling, S.A., Paykel, E.S., Dunn, V.J., Abbott, R. and Katona, C. (2000) Long-term outcome of severe puerperal psychiatric illness: a 23 year follow-up study. *Psychological Medicine*, **30**, 1263–1271.

Rokach, A. (2004) Giving life: loneliness, pregnancy and motherhood. *Social Behaviour and Personality: An International Journal*, **32** (7), 691–702.

Royal College of Physicians (2004) *Briefing on Women in Medicine.* http://www.rcplondon.ac.uk/college/statements/briefing_womenmed.asp (accessed January 2007).

Ryding, E., Wijma, B. and Wijma, K. (1997) Post traumatic stress reactions after emergency caesarean section. *Acta Obstetrica et Gynaecologica Scandinavica,* **76**, 856–861.

Saisto, T., Salmela-Aro, K., Nurmi, J.-E., Kononen, T. and Halmesmaki, E. (2001) A randomized controlled trial of intervention in fear of childbirth. *Obstetrics and Gynecology,* **98**, 820–826.

Schopf, J. and Rust, B. (1994) Follow-up and family study of postpartum psychoses. Part 1: overview. *European Archives of Psychiatry and Clinical Neuroscience,* **244**, 101–111.

Seguin, L. (1999) Depressive symptoms in the late postpartum among low socio-economic status women. *Birth,* **26** (3), 157–163.

Seyfried, L. and Marcus, M. (2003) Postpartum mood disorders. *International Review of Psychiatry,* **15** (3), 231–242.

SIGN (2002) *Postnatal Depression and Puerperal Psychosis.* Scottish Intercollegiate Guidelines Network, Edinburgh.

Smart, C. (1996) Deconstructing motherhood. In *Good Enough Mothering: Feminist Perspectives on Lone Motherhood* (ed E. Bortolaia Silva). Routledge, London.

Snow, S. (2006) *'Travelling Down the Road Together': Women's Experiences of Student Midwife Care* (unpublished MSc dissertation).

Spielberger, C. (1983) *Manual for the State-Trait Anxiety Inventory (STAI).* Consulting Psychologists Press, California.

Suleiman, S. (1985) Writing and motherhood. In *The [M]other Tongue: Essays in Feminist Psychoanalytic Interpretation* (eds S. Garner, C. Kahane, M. Sprengnether). Cornell University Press, Ithaca.

Treadway, C., Kane, F., Jarrahi-Zadeh, A. and Lipton, M. (1969) A psychoendocrine study of pregnancy and the puerperium. *American Journal of Psychiatry,* **125**, 1380–1386. Cited in Brockington, I. (1996) *Motherhood and Mental Health.* Oxford University Press, Oxford.

Wagner, M. (2002) Fish can't see water: the need to humanize birth. *MIDIRS Midwifery Digest,* **12** (2), 213–220.

Walsh, D. (2002) Fear of labour and birth. *British Journal of Midwifery,* **10** (2), 78.

White, T., Matthey, S., Boyd, K. and Barnett, B. (2006) Postnatal depression and post-traumatic stress after childbirth: prevalence, course and co-occurrence. *Journal of Reproductive and Infant Psychology,* **24** (2), 107–120.

Wiggins, M., Oakley, A., Roberts, I., et al. (2004) The Social Support and Family Health Study: a randomised controlled trial and economic evaluation of two alternative forms of postnatal support for mothers living in disadvantaged inner-city areas. *Health Technology Assessment,* **8**, 32.

Wilson, L., Reid, A., Midmer, D., Biringer, A., Carroll, J. and Stewart, D. (1996) Antenatal psychosocial risk factors associated with adverse postnatal family outcomes. *Canadian Medical Association Journal,* **154**, 785–799.

10
Supporting pregnant women living with HIV

Carolyn Roth and Judith Sunderland

'Those people who were marginalised, stigmatized and discriminated against before HIV arrived – have later become, over time, those at highest risk of HIV infection'. Mann and Tarantola (1996: 463)

This chapter will consider the particular needs of childbearing women who are infected with human immunodeficiency virus (HIV) and the role of the community midwife in caring for these women. Community midwives are likely to encounter women with HIV who have been diagnosed during the current pregnancy or who knew their HIV status prior to conception and it is incumbent upon them to acquire sufficient knowledge to be able to respond appropriately to the needs of this client group.

While the pregnant woman with HIV requires the same care and attention as every other pregnant woman, there are particular considerations for her care. These include measures to reduce the risk of mother-to-child transmission (MTCT) of HIV, the need for medication during pregnancy and for the baby after birth, and decision making around the mode of delivery and avoidance of breastfeeding. The community midwife needs to be knowledgeable about these interventions, whether she/he is providing care for a woman throughout her pregnancy or only meets her in the postnatal period. In some respects the role of the community midwife will be to complement, continue and support the advice and treatment that the woman will be receiving from HIV specialist professionals. To do this effectively, she requires a sound knowledge and awareness of local policies and procedures as well as the woman's care plan, treatment and arrangements for follow-up of the woman and her baby. She/he will also need to be familiar with the pathways of communication to key members of the wider HIV team.

Global patterns of HIV infection

In 2005, it was estimated that between 33.4 and 46.0 million people worldwide were living with HIV. Approximately 4.1 million people were newly infected in that year and about 2.8 million people died as a consequence of HIV infection.

In recent years, women have constituted a growing proportion of people living with HIV. In 1997, women represented 41% of people with HIV, and this rose to nearly 50% in 2002. This rise is most marked in the parts of the world where heterosexual transmission is predominant, particularly the Caribbean and sub-Saharan Africa. In addition, women are also represented in epidemics associated with injecting drug use, mobile populations and prisoners (UNAIDS, 2004).

Women are specifically vulnerable to acquiring HIV for reasons that range from the biological to the social, cultural and economic. When acquired immune deficiency syndrome (AIDS) first emerged as a major public health issue in the early 1980s, its significance for women and for pregnancy was not immediately apparent. The first case of AIDS in a child was recognised in 1982, 18 months after the recognition of AIDS in adults. This led to the subsequent implementation of research programmes during the 1980s that identified the pattern of maternal transmission to the fetus and newborn (Mofenson, 1997).

Men can transmit HIV to women much more efficiently than women can to men (European Study Group on Heterosexual Transmission of HIV, 1992). Anatomically, the greater surface area of the female genital tract and the potential for minor degrees of tissue damage increases women's' vulnerability to sexually transmitted infections (STIs) and the acquisition of HIV. There is some evidence that the anatomical and immunological changes of pregnancy increase vulnerability to other genital infections (Brunham et al., 1990) and the risk of being infected with HIV is greater if a woman is already infected with another STI. Due to the fact that many STIs are asymptomatic in women, and therefore go untreated, the risk of HIV infection may be increased even more.

Women's ability to negotiate safer sexual practices is also often limited. To date, the best means of barrier protection remains the male condom, the use of which is not fully within a woman's control. In addition, a woman's access to safe sexual practice is inextricably linked to her economic independence. If she is dependent on a man for her housing and livelihood, her capacity to negotiate within an equal sexual relationship may be compromised. Many women are at risk of gender violence and rape within their domestic relationships (Dunkle et al., 2004). Women who become migrants as a consequence of forced migration associated with war, political oppression or dispossession are subject to conditions that predispose to the transmission of HIV, including instability of family relationships and poverty (Maharaj, 1996).

In 2004, there were 2720 new cases of HIV diagnosed in women in the UK (HPA, 2005), compared to 640 in 1997. Most infections were acquired through sexual transmission and three-quarters of the women were probably infected in Africa (UK Collaborative Group for HIV & STI Surveillance, 2005). The rise in diagnoses probably represents not only an increase in infection rates, but also an increase in the numbers of infected women tested for HIV.

Incidence and prevalence of HIV amongst women in the UK

Monitoring the prevalence (i.e. the number of infected people in a given population) of HIV in the UK is based on data from the Unlinked Anonymous Seroprevalence Survey (UASPS). This survey began in 1990 and is now carried out by the Health Protection Agency (HPA). It involves the testing of anonymised blood samples for HIV. The samples are drawn from those that have been collected for other investigations, such as rubella screening, but for which permission has been given by the individual for inclusion in the survey. The rationale for the survey is to measure the distribution of infection, and HIV in particular, in accessible groups of the population. These groups include pregnant women, women having terminations of pregnancy and newborn babies. Amongst women having terminations of pregnancy in the six sentinel centres in London included in the survey, HIV prevalence rose from 1.02% in 2000 to 1.19% in 2004, and was higher than the rate of infection in women continuing their pregnancies and giving birth. Among pregnant women attending for antenatal care in the same six London centres, the prevalence was 0.62% in 2004 (UK Collaborative Group for HIV & STI Surveillance, 2005).

The key source of data relating to prevalence in women giving birth is the anonymous testing of residual neonatal blood spots taken for routine screening and this survey includes the regions East Midlands, East of England, London, North West, South East, West Midlands, Yorkshire, Humberside and Scotland (Figure 10.1).

There has been a marked increase in the prevalence of HIV infection in women giving birth (see Figure 10.1). In England, prevalence rose to 0.11% in 2004 from 0.016% in 1997. Prevalence was highest in women born in sub-Saharan Africa; rising from 1.5% in 1997 up to 2.2% in 2004. For women born in the UK prevalence remained low from 1997 to 2003 at 0.3%, but rose to 0.7% in 2004 (Royal College of Paediatrics and Child Health, 2006). The prevalence in London rose from 0.19% in 1997 to 0.45% in 2004 (UK Collaborative Group for HIV & STI Surveillance, 2005).

Pathophysiology of HIV infection

HIV is a retrovirus which uses an enzyme, called reverse transcriptase, to create DNA copies of its RNA genetic material, which are then integrated into the DNA of the host cells. The virus becomes a permanent

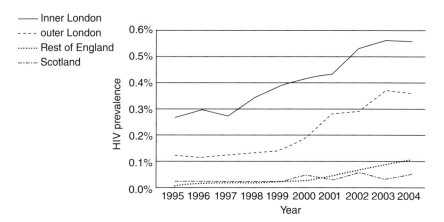

Figure 10.1   HIV prevalence among pregnant women by area of residence. Includes previously diagnosed, those diagnosed through antenatal screening and those remaining undiagnosed. Data source: unlinked anonymous testing of newborn infant dried blood spots. (Reproduced with permission from the Health Protection Agency (HPA, 2005).)

part of the host cells and will replicate itself within them. In the case of HIV, the target cells are those of the immune system. These include CD4 receptors (including T4 helper cells), some macrophages and microglial cells of the brain, amongst others (Pratt, 2003).

The particular part of immune function that is affected is that related to cell-mediated immunity. An infected individual may succumb to a range of infections due to organisms that are widespread within the community but would not ordinarily cause disease in those with intact immune systems. Examples include candida albicans, pneumocystis carinii, herpes zoster and herpes simplex, tuberculosis, cytomegalovirus, toxoplasmosis and some cancers (Pratt, 2003). Women are prone to the same spectrum of opportunistic infections as men, but oesophageal candidiasis, cytomegalovirus disease (CMV) and herpes simplex (HSV) are more common in women than men, while Kaposi's sarcoma is less common in women (Pratt, 2003). HIV also increases the likelihood and severity of a number of gynaecological conditions. These include cervical dysplasia, vulvovaginal candidiasis, pelvic inflammatory disease and prolonged HSV lesions.

Modes of transmission

Although someone infected with HIV often has no signs and symptoms, transmission to another individual is possible at every stage of infection. The primary means of HIV transmission involves direct exposure of mucus membranes to infected blood or other body fluids. This may occur as a result of:

•   sexual contact with an infected person through vaginal or anal intercourse and, possibly, oral exposure to semen or vaginal fluid

- injection of infected blood through the sharing of contaminated injecting equipment (the inadvertent contamination of manufactured blood products or blood transfusion remains a theoretical risk, but in the UK the National Blood Service has implemented measures to reduce the risk to an extremely low level (Stainsby et al., 2005).)
- MTCT, which can occur during the later stages of pregnancy, during a vaginal birth and whilst breastfeeding.

In addition, there is a theoretical risk of infection in the clinical setting due to exposure to specific body fluids, e.g. cerebrospinal fluid, amniotic fluid. Body fluids can also be contaminated by blood as a result of a splash exposure. HIV, however, is a fragile virus that relies on its host for survival and does not survive well outside the body. The likelihood of transmission is dependent upon a number of factors. These include the amount of virus present in the circulation of the infected person to which the recipient is exposed and the way in which exposure occurs, e.g. by injection, blood transfusion, splash exposure or sexual intercourse.

As in the care of all clients, measures must be taken to minimise the possibility of exposure of healthcare workers to blood and other body fluids that may be the source of infective agents including HIV. These precautions also protect the public from exposure to infected staff. Midwives must be familiar with such precautions and should apply these universally (Box 10.1).

Box 10.1 General measures to reduce the risk of occupational exposure

The following measures will help to minimise the risk of exposure to blood-borne viruses and are appropriate for all health settings:

- Wash hands before and after contact with each patient, and before putting on and after removing gloves.
- Change gloves between patients.
- Cover existing wounds, skin lesions and all breaks in exposed skin with waterproof dressings. Wear gloves if hands are extensively affected.
- Wear gloves where contact with blood can be anticipated.
- Avoid sharps usage where possible, and where sharps usage is essential, exercise particular care in handling and disposal.
- Avoid wearing open footwear in situations where blood may be spilt, or where sharp instruments or needles are handled.
- Clear up spillages of blood promptly and disinfect surfaces.
- Wear gloves when cleaning equipment prior to sterilisation or disinfection, when handling chemical disinfectant and when cleaning up spillages.
- Follow safe procedures for disposal of contaminated waste.

Expert Advisory Group on AIDS and the Advisory Group on Hepatitis (1998). Crown Copyright.

Any additional precautions taken in the care of an HIV positive woman are unnecessary and risk contributing to stigma and distress for the woman. Midwives should be familiar with local procedures to deal with accidental exposure to blood and body fluids, and should follow these accordingly.

Natural history of HIV infection

Initial infection with HIV often does not give rise to obvious signs and symptoms. The immune system can remain uncompromised for up to 10 years after the initial infection. Occasionally, the newly infected person will experience a transient flu-like illness, characterised by general malaise, pyrexia and lymphadenopathy (Pratt, 2003).

Clinical signs and symptoms will present due to the opportunistic infections, acquired when the immune system of the HIV-infected person becomes compromised. Signs and symptoms will vary depending on the extent of immune compromise and the particular opportunistic infections involved (Box 10.2).

Box 10.2 WHO staging system for HIV infection and disease in adults and adolescents

Clinical stage I

1. Asymptomatic
2. Persistent generalised lymphadenopathy

Performance scale 1: asymptomatic, normal activity

Clinical stage II

3. Weight loss <10% of body weight
4. Minor mucocutaneous manifestations (seborrheic dermatitis, prurigo, fungal nail infections, recurrent oral ulcerations, angular cheilitis)
5. *Herpes zoster* within the last 5 years
6. Recurrent upper respiratory tract infections (i.e. bacterial sinusitis)

And/or performance scale 2: symptomatic, normal activity

Clinical stage III

7. Weight loss >10% of body weight
8. Unexplained chronic diarrhoea >1 month
9. Unexplained prolonged fever (intermittent or constant) >1 month
10. Oral candidiasis (thrush)
11. Oral hairy leukoplakia

Continued

12. Pulmonary tuberculosis within the past year
13. Severe bacterial infections (i.e. pneumonia, pyomyositis)

And/or performance scale 3: bedridden <50% of the day during the last month

Clinical stage IV

14. HIV wasting syndrome, as defined by the Centers for Disease Control and Prevention
15. *Pneumocystis carinii* pneumonia
16. Toxoplasmosis of the brain
17. Cryptosporidiosis with diarrhoea >1 month
18. Cryptococcosis, extrapulmonary
19. Cytomegalovirus disease of an organ other than liver, spleen or lymph nodes
20. Herpes simplex virus infection, mucocutaneous >1 month or visceral any duration
21. Progressive multifocal leukoencephalopathy
22. Any disseminated endemic mycosis (i.e. histoplasmosis, coccidioidomycosis)
23. Candidiasis of the oesophagus, trachea, bronchi or lungs
24. Atypical mycobacteriosis, disseminated
25. Non-typhoid *Salmonella* septicaemia
26. Extrapulmonary tuberculosis
27. Lymphoma
28. Kaposi's sarcoma
29. HIV encephalopathy, as defined by the Centers for Disease Control and Prevention.

And/or performance scale 4: bedridden >50% of the day during the last month

Reproduced with permission from the World Health Organization. http://www. unaids.org/en/MediaCentre/References/default.asp#begin (accessed 16.2.07).

Screening for HIV in pregnancy

The current approach to HIV in pregnancy in the UK is built on three key objectives: diagnosis before or during pregnancy, management of maternal HIV disease as appropriate and measures to reduce MTCT.

Diagnosis

Women can be diagnosed with HIV prior to, during or after pregnancy. HIV testing may be undertaken when:

- a woman believes that she has been exposed to the virus due to a diagnosis of HIV, or illness, in a sexual partner
- a woman has symptoms suggestive of opportunistic infection or immune compromise
- screening is offered as an integral part of routine antenatal care
- a diagnosis of HIV infection in a woman's baby has been confirmed.

Women will only be in a position of being able to choose interventions to prevent neonatal infection, and to reduce the impact of HIV infection on their own health, if they are aware of their own HIV status. Recommendations to support routine antenatal screening were put forward by the Royal College of Paediatrics and Child Health (1998) and the DH (1999) and implemented in 2000. Antenatal HIV testing is offered and recommended to all women attending for antenatal care. If the initial visit for antenatal care is conducted in the community, it will be the responsibility of the community midwife to explain the rationale for testing and to seek the woman's consent (Box 10.3).

Box 10.3 Practice point: routine screening for HIV

- When presenting the test it is important to remain unbiased.
- Emphasise the benefits of early diagnosis for women's health and reduction of MTCT.
- It is good practice to support this discussion with written information.

The emerging outcome of universal antenatal HIV testing is that pregnant women most commonly discover their HIV infection as a result of antenatal HIV testing. Whereas in 1997 only one-third of the 300 HIV-infected women giving birth were diagnosed prior to delivery, more than 90% of 1000 affected pregnant women were diagnosed prior to the birth of their babies in 2004 (Figure 10.2). However, although the proportion of infection in the exposed newborn has reduced, the numbers of infected babies born overall has not declined (Royal College of Paediatrics and Child Health, 2006). All of these factors confirm the importance of midwives' awareness and knowledge of HIV in order to provide the best care for women.

HIV is diagnosed on the basis of testing the blood for antibodies to the virus. Diagnosis of HIV always relies on at least two tests. The first is the enzyme linked immunoassay test (ELISA). This is a highly sensitive test that detects the presence of HIV antibodies but, because of its sensitivity, it may sometimes become positive because of the presence of antibodies to other viruses (false positive). Therefore, when this test is positive, the blood sample is also tested by means of the Western Blot, a test with a higher specificity for HIV antibodies. The Western Blot test uses chromatography to identify the presence of HIV antibodies and has a very low false positive rate. The combination of these two

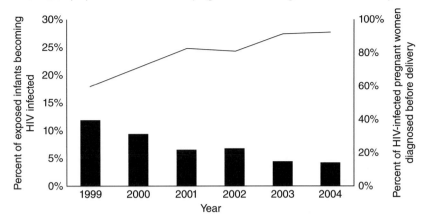

Figure 10.2 Proportion of HIV-infected women diagnosed before the birth of their babies. Includes previously diagnosed and those diagnosed through antenatal testing. (Reproduced with permission from the Health Protection Agency (HPA, 2005).)

tests increases the reliability of diagnosis. Occasionally, the test results are reported as 'indeterminate', in which case it is likely that a second blood sample will need to be collected to confirm the results.

Disclosing the diagnosis

Informing women of their HIV positive status in pregnancy requires a balance between acknowledging the impact of the diagnosis on the woman and the need to impart specific information concerning her health needs and those of her baby. Because of the nature and volume of information to be conveyed and the emotional impact of the diagnosis, the process should be paced to take into account the woman's ability to absorb new information and its relevance at different stages of pregnancy. This should be undertaken by someone with a very good knowledge of the implications of HIV infection in pregnant women, who has the confidence and experience to discuss sensitive issues. In areas where there has been limited experience in the care of HIV positive women, the most appropriate person may not be a midwife, but rather a member of the sexual health team. However, it is important that a midwife be involved at the earliest stages in order to gain that experience and to offer ongoing care to the woman and her family.

Great consideration must be given to how and when the woman is invited to receive her results. Midwives should be aware of local policy. This should take into account protection of the woman's confidentiality and the availability of support (Box 10.4).

Box 10.4 Practice point: disclosure of diagnosis

- It is good practice for women to be invited to discuss the results of their blood tests by a letter, rather than telephone.
- Avoid any reference to the HIV test until the face-to-face discussion takes place.
- The meeting should take place in a room which affords privacy and no likelihood of interruption.
- Never give results late in the day or at the end of the week – this would limit easy access to further information and support should the woman need it immediately following diagnosis.
- Once the results have been discussed with the woman, check with her to find out whether there is someone she would like to contact to come to meet her at the clinic.
- Provide all women with the contact telephone number of a designated person who will be available to answer further questions when they arise.

Many women affected by HIV are from migrant communities and therefore may not have English as their first language. It is essential that provision for advocacy or interpreting be available when these women are given their results and at all subsequent visits for care.

Monitoring and treatment

Once a diagnosis of HIV has been confirmed, a number of investigations are employed to ascertain the status of the infection. The viral load is measured to determine the quantity of circulating virus in the blood and this is expressed as copies of the virus per millilitre of blood. In addition, the CD4 count is measured as a reflection of the impact of the virus on the immune system. The normal range for a CD4 count in a healthy adult is between 500 and 1500 cells/mm^3. In addition, clinical examination will be undertaken to detect HIV-associated signs such as oral hairy leucoplakia, lymphadenopathy, oral or ano-genital candidiasis.

Decisions about drug treatment will be made depending on the results of these investigations. Not all individuals diagnosed with HIV will require treatment at the time of diagnosis. If the infected person is asymptomatic, the decision will be made primarily on the basis of their CD4 count. When this is between 200 and 350 cells/mm^3 then the initiation of treatment is likely to be advised. If the individual is symptomatic, there will usually be an associated CD4 count of less than 350 cells/mm^3. However, initiation of treatment would be suggested regardless of the CD4 count (BHIVA, 2005a). Other data, such as viral load, will also be taken into account to guide management decisions. In the case of pregnancy, there are additional considerations regarding the choice of drugs and the timing of the initiation of treatment. A detailed discussion of relevant considerations can be found in the British HIV Association (BHIVA) guidelines (BHIVA, 2005b).

Medication for HIV infection in pregnancy has two separate objectives: to reduce MTCT and to treat the woman's HIV disease itself, if that is required. Some form of antiretroviral therapy will be suggested to all women who are diagnosed with HIV during pregnancy, with the aim of making transmission of HIV to the baby less likely and optimising the woman's own health.

Monotherapy with zidovudine (ZDV) is likely to be suggested if a woman has a viral load of less than 6–10 000 HIV RNA copies/ml plasma, does not require highly active antiretroviral therapy (HAART) for her own HIV infection, or does not wish to take it and is willing to have a planned caesarean for delivery (BHIVA, 2005b).

For a newly diagnosed woman with a viral load of more than 10 000 HIV RNA copies/ml plasma or signs of immune compromise, a combination of antiretroviral drugs will be recommended because of the need for treatment of her own infection, in addition to preventing MTCT. Because of the large variety of available drugs and the considerations relevant to individual women, these treatment decisions are complex. The principles guiding decision-making are to achieve a balance between optimal maternal health with minimal risk of drug exposure to the fetus. For specific illustrations of treatment decisions refer to the BHIVA guidelines (BHIVA, 2005b).

Some women will already be taking medication at the time of conception and in most cases will continue with the same medication. Occasionally, the choice of drugs might be adjusted to achieve the principles identified above.

Prevention of mother to child transmission

In the absence of maternal antiretroviral therapy during pregnancy, approximately 1 in 7 babies born to HIV infected women will be born with HIV infection. Since the introduction of antiretroviral therapy (ART) in 1987 for individuals with HIV infection its efficacy in reducing MTCT in pregnancy has been proven (Connor et al., 1994). The prognosis for HIV-infected women and their babies has improved significantly. It is, however, important to be aware that availability of ART is limited in the parts of the world where HIV is most prevalent, and therefore the consequences of HIV infection for women and their babies vary according to where they live, how much money they have and the accessibility to medical care (McIntyre, 2005).

As knowledge and understanding of MTCT have increased, a number of strategies have been implemented to reduce the likelihood of perinatal infection. These include choosing caesarean section as the mode of birth and the avoidance of prolonged rupture of membranes, prolonged labour and breastfeeding (Brocklehurst and Volminck, 2002). With the increased use of HAART during pregnancy, which suppresses the amount of maternal circulating virus, the role of planned elective caesarean section is currently being reconsidered (BHIVA, 2005b; Read and Newell, 2005).

The most significant intervention aiming to reduce the incidence of MTCT has been associated with the use of the drug ZDV. The AIDS Clinical Trial Group study 076 demonstrated that when ZDV was taken by the woman from the second trimester onwards and given to babies for 6 weeks after birth, transmission of HIV to the newborn was reduced by two-thirds from 25 to 8.4% (Connor et al., 1994).

Currently, newborns in the UK will be prescribed ZDV for approximately 4 weeks as an additional protection against infection due to exposure at the time of birth. In some cases, the baby may be prescribed an alternative antiretroviral regime if, for example, maternal viral load was unknown or detectable at the time of delivery or if ZDV was contraindicated for the mother during pregnancy (Box 10.5).

Box 10.5 Practice point: fetal and neonatal health

There are additional concerns that community midwives need to be aware of when monitoring fetal growth and neonatal health.

- There is evidence that intrauterine growth restriction and preterm labour are both more common in the pregnancies of HIV-infected women. Ellis et al. (2002) demonstrated a greater incidence of low birth weight and preterm delivery in untreated HIV-infected women in an inner city setting in the USA.
- There is also some evidence from the ongoing European Collaborative Study that there is a higher rate of prematurity and severe prematurity in babies born to women treated with HAART (Thorne et al., 2004).
- Women who are immuno-compromised will have a predisposition to HSV and CMV, both of which can be transmitted to the neonate. This has clear implications for neonatal health because these viruses are associated with severe, overwhelming infection in the newborn.

Infant feeding

The decision about infant feeding will be an important aspect of ante-natal discussion because the risk of transmission from breastfeeding is significant and bottlefeeding is strongly recommended (Dunn et al.,

1992). Many women will face a real dilemma. Not only will they be disappointed to discover that breastfeeding may place their child at risk, but they may also have to identify the fact that by not breastfeeding their baby there is the potential for unintended disclosure of their HIV status. This can be a source of great difficulty for women who have not disclosed their status to partners, family and friends. They may have to provide explanations concerning the method of feeding they are using, particularly when breastfeeding is a cultural norm within the woman's community. Women will need to consider how they may react when faced with disapproval or questions from partner, family, friends and the wider community. It is particularly important to avoid a situation in which a woman feels pressured to breastfeed in order to avoid answering the uncomfortable questions that may be raised by her partner and family. This could give rise to mixed feeding, e.g. offering the baby both breast milk and formula milk, which evidence suggests may facilitate HIV transmission (Coutsoudis et al., 2001).

Suppression of lactation with an appropriate drug after the birth is one option that the midwife can explore with the woman. The avoidance of not only the physical discomfort of engorged breasts but also the reminder of having to avoid breastfeeding may be right for some women. The availability of lactation suppressants can be discussed and arranged before birth.

It is vital that midwives recognise the crucial links highlighted above. Emphasis must be placed upon the fact that a discussion about infant feeding is also a discussion about her feelings regarding disclosure of her HIV status and how she might approach this.

Disclosure to family and friends

The level of stigma that continues to surround HIV in the UK may be compounded by the woman's experience of HIV in her country of origin. HIV has a different meaning in a resource poor setting, compared to the developed world where treatment is both free and available (Moore et al., 2002). A woman's fear of the consequences of disclosure of her HIV status can lead to isolation and the burden of living with secrets. Many women fear that disclosure itself can lead to domestic violence and abandonment. Medley et al.'s (2004) literature review about disclosure of HIV status by women in developing countries found that the barriers to disclosure included fear of accusations of infidelity, abandonment, discrimination and violence.

In the early days of diagnosis, a woman can feel that disclosure of her HIV status is just not possible. Readiness to disclose HIV status is a process rather than a single event and she may need time to achieve this (Holt et al., 1998). It is not unusual to find that disclosure has not occurred before the birth of the baby. Both community- and hospital-based midwives need to be very aware of where the woman has reached in disclosing to relatives, as the need to protect her confidentiality may be an issue during her postnatal care. Questions are likely to arise from relatives about the reason for caesarean section, medication of the baby and bottle feeding. The community midwife has an important role in discussing with the woman, in advance, how she would like these issues to be handled.

There is an increasing number of HIV positive women who embark on a pregnancy and who may have been living with their HIV diagnosis for some time. They may already have started to come to terms with their diagnosis, be established on ART and worked through issues of disclosure. However, many of the issues discussed above will still be pertinent in planning their midwifery care.

Emerging issues

The shock of diagnosis during pregnancy will give rise to a great deal of anxiety for a woman in relation to her current and future health, the risks to her unborn baby, and the likelihood of her partner or other children also having the virus. HIV-positive pregnant women will also need to make certain key decisions within a time frame dictated by the pregnancy. If she has booked late and/or has been diagnosed late in her pregnancy, this time frame will be considerably reduced and the pressure on her to make decisions and her need for support will be more urgent.

Concerns about her own health and transmission to the unborn baby will be addressed by referral to an HIV physician, who will do a full assessment to determine the stage of maternal infection and the need for treatment.

The infection status of her partner and other children will need to be discussed. Following an unexpected diagnosis of HIV during pregnancy, it is likely that a woman will require extensive support and a period of time before she is ready to share this with her partner. Her partner may already be infected but not tested or he may be free of infection but at risk of becoming infected as a consequence of unprotected sexual intercourse. Thus, the issues she may need to discuss will include disclosure to her partner and the availability of testing for her partner. She should also be given information about using condoms to reduce the risk of transmission, although this will require her to talk with him about her diagnosis, which she may not feel is immediately possible.

She is also likely to be fearful about the possibility of having acquired the infection prior to earlier pregnancies and the risk of exposure of her older children. It is extremely important that there is an opportunity for the woman to discuss whether and when to have them tested for HIV and a paediatrician should be involved in dialogue as a matter of course. It is important to bear in mind the immense impact if others within the family are diagnosed around the same time and appropriate multi-agency support should be facilitated.

Continuing care

Continuity of care from a single known midwife will be especially important for the woman who is HIV positive. This will ensure consistency of information and avoids the need for her to re-tell her story to many different people. The midwife providing care may be someone with a special remit for the care of an HIV positive woman, but this is dependent on local resources and needs. However, the maternity unit should develop links with local sexual health services so that information and support for the midwife is available if required. If possible the continuity of midwifery care should extend into the postnatal period. Other professionals, for example the community midwife, health visitor and GP should, with the woman's permission, be included in this communication of information to ensure that advice is accurate and consistent. Maintaining confidentiality is of the utmost importance and sharing of information between colleagues must only be done to enhance communication. The rationale for professionals to be made aware of a woman's HIV status is the facilitation of effective care and for no other reason.

Women should be informed about community-based HIV organisations (e.g. Positively Women or Terrence Higgins Trust) who offer information and one-to-one peer support. In addition, it is important to give the woman information about support organisations in her area of residence. This information will be available from the local sexual health/HIV clinic.

Coordination of services

A number of different professionals will be involved in a woman's care and the coordination of services will be essential for optimal benefit and to avoid inconvenience, confusion and conflicting advice. This role would be appropriately undertaken by the midwife. In addition to the care and support of the midwife and advocate/ interpreter, every woman should be referred to an obstetrician, an HIV physician, counsellor or health advisor, paediatrician, HIV clinical nurse specialist and, if required, a social worker. While the majority of the woman's HIV care will be undertaken by a physician with specialist knowledge of HIV, it is important to acknowledge the contribution of her GP as part of the primary healthcare team.

The specialist physician will continue to manage the care of the woman after the pregnancy.

In areas of low prevalence of HIV infection, where a positive diagnosis may be infrequent, it is important that referral pathways exist in order to manage the diagnosis, care and follow-up of HIV positive women and their babies. Local arrangements are likely to vary, but everyone involved in antenatal HIV screening should be aware of the mechanisms identified for HIV positive women.

Planning the birth

Community midwives may not be involved in the care of the woman during the birth of the baby but they will be involved in discussing the woman's plans. An awareness of the implications of HIV positive status around the time of birth is therefore necessary if the midwife is going to be able to support the woman in exploring possible options. The key principles informing care for women and babies at the time of birth are:

* Support the woman in achieving the best birth experience possible.
* Take appropriate measures to minimise exposure of the fetus/newborn baby to HIV virus.
* Avoid an exclusive focus upon HIV status at the expense of holistic, woman-centred care.

It is important that plans for the mode of birth and the woman's preferences are discussed at the earliest opportunity and that the discussion is revisited as the pregnancy progresses. A birth plan should be drawn up with the woman that reflects the intended mode of birth and the care she will require. Clear documentation must indicate the actions to be initiated in the event of pre-labour rupture of membranes, the onset of labour prior to a planned date for caesarean section or admission to hospital in spontaneous labour at term. Some maternity units have overcome the potential threats to confidentiality by asking the woman to hand in this care plan when she arrives at the maternity unit.

If the plan is for elective caesarean section and the woman is admitted either in labour or with spontaneous rupture of membranes, a decision about the mode of birth will need to be made urgently by the obstetrician, in consultation with the HIV physician. Intervention should be undertaken at the earliest opportunity as the risk of MTCT increases with the length of time of ruptured membranes (The International Perinatal HIV Group, 2001) (Box 10.6).

Box 10.6 Practice point: labour and birth

- If a vaginal birth is planned, invasive procedures such as artificial rupture of membranes, application of a fetal scalp electrode, fetal blood sampling and episiotomy must be avoided.
- If fetal compromise is identified in labour then emergency caesarean section is the appropriate course of action (BHIVA, 2005b).
- At the time of birth, even if the birth has been by caesarean section and the plan of care is to feed the baby artificially, make sure that the woman and her baby do not miss out on the usual midwifery intervention of early skin-to-skin contact to promote attachment and regulation of the neonate's temperature and respiration.

Neonatal care, testing and follow-up

Current recommendations are that the baby receives oral ZDV (2 mg/kg) twice a day for 4 weeks, ideally commencing within 12 hours of birth (BHIVA, 2005b). It is important to make sure that the woman feels confident about administering the baby's medication prior to going home.

All babies of HIV positive mothers will have circulating HIV antibodies acquired through placental transfer from the mother. This does not mean that the baby is infected with HIV. The antibodies acquired from the mother may persist for up to 18 months after birth. For this reason, the basis for diagnosis of HIV in the newborn is the presence of HIV DNA in the blood. Testing of the newborn for HIV uses polymerase chain reaction (PCR) or other method, to amplify HIV DNA in a peripheral blood sample (BHIVA, 2005b). Since the most likely time of infection is during labour and delivery, levels of HIV DNA may be very low but by 3 months of age, more than 95% of non-breastfed, HIV infected infants will be detected by this method (BHIVA, 2005b). In addition, the use of ZDV or other prophylactic antiretrovirals may alter the result.

BHIVA guidelines recommend that testing be undertaken at 1 day, 6 weeks and 12 weeks of age in order to test the baby after cessation of prophylactic medication. The baby will be considered to be uninfected if all these tests are negative. The uninfected status will be confirmed at 18 months of age if an antibody test is negative. Testing will take place in the paediatric HIV clinic or its equivalent and the appointment for testing at 6 weeks should be made before the woman and baby are discharged from hospital into the community.

It is important to know that the results of these tests can take as long as 6 weeks to be reported. This will clearly be a period of extreme anxiety for the woman and her family. Ideally, the clinical nurse specialist will be visiting the woman at home to offer support in addition to postnatal visits from the community midwife and home visits from the health visitor. The paediatric team with responsibility for HIV care will convey the results of neonatal testing and provide continuing care should a diagnosis of HIV be made.

Monitoring of pregnancies with HIV, transmission and treatment effects

Clinicians caring for women with HIV and their children are encouraged to report new pregnancies to the UK National Study of HIV in Pregnancy (NSHPC), which has collected data on pregnancy outcomes associated with HIV since June 1989 (Tookey, 2005). In addition, clinical details of women receiving ART will be reported to the International Drug Registry antenatally, and infants to the British Paediatric Surveillance Unit (BPSU) after birth. Long-term follow-up of ART exposed infants is being undertaken via the Children exposed to ART (CHART) study (Hankins et al., 2004).

Case study 10.1 offers you the opportunity to investigate the journey of an HIV-positive pregnant woman from diagnosis to postnatal care in your locality. You are probably aware of some local arrangements but it will be useful for you to enquire about policies, protocols and personnel involved in planning and delivering HIV services.

Case study 10.1 Sarah's case

You met Sarah at 12 weeks in her first pregnancy. During the booking interview, you obtained her consent for all the antenatal blood tests, including HIV antibody testing. Today you received notification from the virology laboratory that her HIV antibody test is positive.

- What local arrangements exist in your practice setting for informing women of a positive HIV antibody result?
- Who is expected to inform Sarah of her results?
- How will Sarah be contacted about the appointment?
- Where will the consultation take place?

- Who will support Sarah around the issue of disclosure of her diagnosis to her partner?
- Where would Sarah's partner be able to be tested for HIV antibodies, if he so chooses?
- Who takes the lead for the clinical care of individuals with HIV in pregnancy?
- How will Sarah's ongoing care for HIV infection be organised and managed?
- What sources of support for HIV positive women exist in your area and how will you ensure that Sarah knows about them?
- What arrangements will be made for her midwifery/obstetric care during this pregnancy?
- Who is responsible for coordinating Sarah's care so that her needs arising from HIV infection, in relation to her pregnancy, are fully addressed?
- What clinical care will be provided by the HIV physician/nurses and/or sexual health clinic?
- How can this be organised to avoid unnecessary visits and to keep appointments to the minimum?
- What is the local policy concerning planning mode of delivery for the HIV positive woman?
- When does this discussion take place and who is involved?
- If a decision has been made with Sarah for elective caesarean section, in the event of the onset of spontaneous labour how will the delivery be managed?
- Who will be responsible for coordinating Sarah and her baby's transfer from hospital and her continuing care?
- What information will be provided to the community midwife, health visitor and GP?
- Who will discuss this transfer of information with Sarah?
- What arrangements are there in your area for follow-up of Sarah's baby?

Summary

This chapter has provided an overview of the main issues that emerge for women diagnosed with HIV infection during pregnancy. Women who are HIV positive and pregnant have to confront a multitude of challenges. They will be best served by midwives who are well-informed, non-judgemental, flexible and able to respond to each woman as an individual.

⟨◻⟩⟶   **Key points**

- Antenatal screening for HIV has made an important contribution in reducing infant HIV infection and should be recommended for all pregnant women.
- Women must have information about antenatal screening that is informative, unbiased and easily understood, and they must be allowed adequate time to make a decision to be tested.
- Each maternity unit should have policies and protocols outlining the care of pregnant women with a positive HIV result.
- Each maternity unit should have at least one member of staff who is able to give women an HIV diagnosis. That person must have knowledge about HIV in pregnancy and its treatment, awareness of the range of women's responses to HIV diagnosis, and familiarity with local referral pathways for both the woman and her family.
- Following diagnosis women should have a named member of staff who can explain their treatment, answer their questions and provide continuity of care.
- Women should be informed about local and national support networks.
- Women with HIV infection have the right to expect excellence in the care they receive for both their pregnancy and HIV, whatever the care setting.

References

BHIVA (2005a) *The British HIV Association Guidelines for the Treatment of HIV-Infected Adults with Antiretroviral Therapy.* http://www.bhiva.org/index.html.

BHIVA (2005b) *Guidelines for the Management of HIV infection in Pregnant Women and the Prevention of Mother-to-Child Transmission of HIV.* http://www.bhiva.org/index.html.

Brocklehurst, P. and Volminck, J. (2002) Antiretrovirals for reducing the risk of mother-to-child transmission of HIV infection. *Cochrane Database of Systematic Reviews*, Issue 2. Art. No. CD003510.

Brunham, R.C., Holmes, K.K. and Embree, J.E. (1990) Sexually transmitted diseases in pregnancy. In *Sexually Transmitted Diseases* (eds K.K. Holmes, P.A. Mardh, P.F. Sparling et al.), 2nd edn. McGraw-Hill, New York.

Connor, E.M., Sperling, R.S., Gelber, R., et al. (1994) Reduction of maternal–infant transmission of human immunodeficiency virus type 1 with zidovudine treatment. Pediatric AIDS Clinical Trials Group Protocol 076 Study Group. *New England Journal of Medicine*, **331** (18), 1173–1180.

Coutsoudis, A., Pillay, K., Kuhn, L., et al. (2001) Method of feeding and transmission of HIV from mothers to children by 15 months of age: prospective cohort study from Durban, South Africa. *AIDS*, **15**, 379–387.

DH (1999) *Reducing Mother to Baby Transmission of HIV*. Health Sevice Circular, 1999/183.

Dunkle, K.L., Jewkes, R.K., Brown, H.C., Gray, G.E., McIntyre, J.A. and Harlow, S.D. (2004) Gender-based violence, relationship power, and risk of HIV infection in women attending antenatal clinics in South Africa. *Lancet*, **363** (9419), 1415–1421.

Dunn, D.M., Newell, M.L., Ades, A. and Peckham, C. (1992) Risk of human immunodeficiency virus type – 1 transmission through breast feeding. *Lancet*, **340** (8827), 585–588.

Ellis, J., Williams, H., Graves, W. and Lindsay, M.K. (2002) Human immunodefiency virus infection is a risk factor for adverse perinatal outcome. *American Journal of Obstetrics & Gynaecology*, **186** (5), 903–906.

European Study Group on Heterosexual Transmission of HIV. (1992) Comparison of female-to-male and male-to-female transmission of HIV in 563 stable couples. *British Medical Journal*, **304**, 809–813.

Expert Advisory Group on AIDS and the Advisory Group on Hepatitis (1998). *Guidance for Clinical Health Care Workers: Protection against Infection with Blood-Borne Viruses*. HSC, London. http://www.dh.gov.uk/en/Publicationsandstatistics/Publications/PublicationsPolicyAndGuidance/DH_4002766 (accessed 14.6.07).

Hankins, C.D., Tookey, P.A., Lyall, E.G.H. and Peckham, C.S. (2004) Follow-up of children exposed to antiretroviral therapy in pregnancy (CHART): a role for HIV physicians. *HIV Medicine*, **5** (Suppl 2), 35–36.

Holt, R., Court, P., Vedhara, K., Nott, K.H., Holmes, J. and Snow, M.H. (1998) The role of disclosure in coping with HIV infection. *AIDS Care* **10**, 1.

HPA (2005) *HIV and Other Sexually Transmitted Infections in the UK*. Health Protection Agency, London.

Maharaj, B. (1996) The historical development of the apartheid local state in South Africa: The case of Durban. *International Journal of Urban and Regional Research*, **20** (4), 587–600.

Mann, J. and Tarantola, D.J.M. (1996) *AIDS in the World: Global Dimensions, Social Roots and Responses*, Vol. 2, Oxford University Press, USA.

McIntyre, J. (2005) Maternal health and HIV. *Reproductive Health Matters*, **13** (25), 129–135.

Medley, A., Garcia-Moreno, C., McGill, S. and Maman, S. (2004) Rates, barriers and outcomes of HIV serostatus disclosure among women in developing countries: implications for prevention of mother-to-child transmission programmes. *Bulletin of the World Health Organization*, **82** (4), 299–307.

Mofenson, L.M. (1997) Interaction between timing of perinatal human immunodeficiency virus infection and the design of preventive and therapeutic interventions. *Acta Paediatrica*, **421** (Suppl), 1–9.

Moore, A., Madge, S. and Johnson, M. (2002) HIV in pregnancy. *The Obstetrician and Gynaecologist*, **4** (4), 197–200.

Pratt, R. (2003) *HIV & AIDS: A Strategy for Nursing Care*, 5th edn. Edward Arnold, London.

Read, J.S. and Newell, M.L. (2005) Efficacy and safety of caesarean delivery for prevention of mother-to-child transmission of HIV-1. *The Cochrane Database of Systematic Reviews*, Issue 4, Art. No. CD005479.

Royal College of Paediatrics and Child Health (1998) *Intercollegiate Working Party for Enhancing Voluntary Confidential HIV Testing in Pregnancy*. Royal College of Paediatrics and Child Health, London.

Royal College of Paediatrics and Child Health (2006) *Reducing Mother to Child Transmission of HIV Infection in the United Kingdom: Update Report of an Intercollegiate Working Party*. Royal College of Paediatrics and Child Health, London.

Stainsby, D., Cohen, H., Jones, H., et al. (2005) *Serious Hazards of Transfusion: Annual Report 2004*. Serious Hazards of Transfusion Steering Group, Manchester.

The International Perinatal HIV Group (2001) Duration of ruptured membranes and vertical transmission of HIV-1: a meta-analysis from 15 prospective cohort studies. *AIDS*, **15**, 357–368.

Thorne, C., Patel, D. and Newell, M.L. (2004) Increased risk of adverse pregnancy outcomes in HIV-infected women treated with highly active antiretroviral therapy in Europe. *AIDS*, **18** (17), 2337–2339.

Tookey, P. (2005) *National Study of HIV in Pregnancy & Childhood: RCOG Report*. RCOG, London.

UK Collaborative Group for HIV & STI Surveillance (2005) *Mapping the Issues: HIV and other Sexually Transmitted Infections in the United Kingdom*. Health Protection Agency Centre for Infections, London.

UNAIDS (2004) Fast Facts about AIDS. *http://www.unaids.org/en/MediaCentre/References/default.asp#begin* (accessed 16.2.07).

Domestic abuse: supporting women and asking the question

Ruth Jones

'Audra Bancroft was murdered by her boyfriend, Gary Walker, a policeman, in their flat in Burton-upon-Trent in 2003. She was four months' pregnant, and sustained more than 50 injuries.'
Viner (2005)

'Domestic abuse' is a term that is increasingly being used to define the phenomenon that has historically been referred to as domestic violence, although on the whole official and legal definitions continue to use the term 'domestic violence'.

The government defines domestic violence as 'any incident of threatening behaviour, violence or abuse (psychological, physical, sexual, financial or emotional) between adults who are or have been intimate partners or family members, regardless of gender or sexuality' (DH, 2005).

This definition mirrors that of the Association of Chief Police Officers (which they recommend all police forces use) and attempts to incorporate the continuum of behaviours that constitute domestic violence. In spite of this, the term 'domestic violence' can be problematic as it implies that such violence will be physical in form and will result in physical injury. Findings from Kershaw et al. (2001) show that this is true with injuries often sustained as a result of domestic abuse, especially among women. During the worst incidents of domestic violence experienced in 2001, 46 per cent of women sustained a minor physical injury, 20 per cent a moderate physical injury, and six per cent severe injuries (Walby and Allen, 2004). Statistics also show that there were 116 women killed by current or former partners in 2001/02. This equates to an average of more than two deaths each week (Flood-Page and Taylor, 2003).

Domestic violence is not purely physical. It encompasses a continuum of behaviours, including psychological, emotional, sexual and financial abuse. These behaviours alone, or combined with physical abuse, can have devastating effects, with abused women being 'more likely to suffer from depression, anxiety, psychosomatic symptoms, eating problems and sexual dysfunction' (WHO, 2000). Such effects can be harder to recognise as results of domestic violence and it is consequently more difficult for professionals to respond effectively. The transition in terminology from domestic violence to domestic abuse attempts to highlight the wide range of behaviours that constitute the phenomenon, and aids the recognition of, and responses to, this complex issue.

In Position Paper 19a, *Domestic Abuse in Pregnancy* (RCM, 1999), the Royal College of Midwives (RCM) use the term 'domestic abuse' to describe violence 'perpetrated by an adult against another with whom they have or have had a sexual relationship'. This chapter will follow suit, using the term 'domestic abuse' to discuss the reasons why midwives should raise the question of domestic abuse with the women they meet. It will also address how to do so effectively, whilst considering issues of confidentiality and good practice. When referring to those experiencing such abuse, the focus will be on women, reflecting the fact that research consistently shows that women report more frequent assaults, more severe injuries and are more likely to report fear as a result of domestic violence (Walby and Allen, 2004). And, of course, this chapter relates to domestic abuse during pregnancy.

The evidence base for routine enquiry

There are a number of 'signs' or indicators that may alert a midwife to the existence of domestic abuse. However, the existence of one or more of these does not automatically mean that abuse is occurring, although *Responding to Domestic Abuse: A Handbook for Health Professionals* (DH, 2005) tells us that these signs should raise suspicion and prompt health professionals to ask if the woman is being abused (Box 11.1).

Box 11.1 'Signs' or indicators of domestic abuse

- History of domestic abuse.
- Visible suspicious injuries/injuries inconsistent with explanation.
- Late booking.
- Sporadic utilisation of prenatal care.

Continued

- Multiple visits for vague somatic complaints.
- Frequently missed appointments/cancellation of two or more appointments by a partner.
- History of miscarriage/terminations/still birth/pre-term labour.
- Chronic pain.
- Headache.
- Pelvic or abdominal pain.
- History of repeated frequent vaginal or urinary tract infections.
- Substance misuse.
- Stress-related symptoms such as fatigue, anxiety and difficulty concentrating.
- Eating disorders.
- Depression.
- Suicide attempts.

The term 'selective screening' is used when health professionals question only the women who display such 'signs' of domestic abuse. There has been a lot of debate in recent years about whether health professionals, and midwives in particular, should introduce routine enquiry about domestic abuse (Waalen et al., 2000; Ramsay et al., 2002; Mezey et al., 2003; Taket et al., 2003). Routine enquiry by midwives would mean that all pregnant women would be asked about domestic abuse whether or not they have any signs or indicators that raise concerns.

A strong case exists for routine enquiry because statistics show that one in four women are victims of domestic abuse during their lifetime (Mooney, 1993); in 30% of cases, domestic abuse will occur for the first time during pregnancy and existing abuse will often escalate during pregnancy (McWilliams and McKinnon, 1993; Lewis, 2001; DH, 2005). The reasons for this are varied and complex but can include the added financial difficulties that pregnancy can bring, jealousy, dislike of the pregnant woman's changing body and changes in sexual libido. Whatever the reason might be, it is distressing to identify that what is supposed to be a joyful time instead sees the beginning of a turbulent and potentially dangerous period for these women and their unborn children.

The stress caused to pregnant women as a result of domestic abuse can result in problems during pregnancy (see Box 11.2), such as low weight gain, anaemia, infections and bleeding, and can ultimately cause miscarriage, premature delivery, low birth weight, abruption, stillbirth and maternal death (Newberger et al., 1992; Mezey, 1997; Lewis, 2004).

Box 11.2 Physical effects of abuse during pregnancy

- Insufficient weight gain.
- Anaemia.
- Vaginal/cervical/kidney infections.
- Vaginal bleeding.
- Abdominal trauma.
- Haemorrhage.
- Exacerbation of chronic illnesses.
- Complications during labour.
- Delayed prenatal care.
- Miscarriage.
- Low birth weight.
- Ruptured membranes.
- Placental abruption.
- Uterine infection.
- Fetal bruising, fractures and haematomas.
- Stillbirth.
- Maternal death.

Newberger et al. (1992)

The *Confidential Enquiry into Maternal Deaths* (Lewis, 2004) informs us that 11 women whose deaths were reported to the enquiry were murdered by their partner during pregnancy or within 6 weeks of the birth of their babies, with another being classified as a late death.

The same report tells us that 14% of the 391 women whose deaths were reported to the enquiry had either voluntarily reported domestic abuse to a healthcare professional during their pregnancy or the abuse was already known to be a factor. None had routinely been asked about domestic abuse so this is almost certainly an under-estimate. When we take into consideration that 'the most common cause of indirect deaths and the largest cause of maternal deaths overall was psychiatric illness', a common effect of domestic abuse, coupled with the fact that 30% of domestic abuse begins in pregnancy (McWilliams and McKinnon, 1993; DH, 2005), it seems probable that many more of the women who died were experiencing such abuse.

It may seem shocking that these women did not disclose or were not asked about abuse but as Hegarty et al. tell us 'in contrast to the magnitude of the problem, there is consistent evidence that (a) the majority of women who are being abused by their partner do not disclose this to health professionals and (b) that health professionals are reluctant to inquire about abuse and as a result only a minority of abused women are recognised in health care settings' (Hegarty et al., 2005: 2).

Bacchus et al. (2002) state that routine enquiry about domestic abuse by health professionals in maternity settings is accepted by women, provided it is conducted in a safe and confidential environment. This is backed up by the findings of a pilot project in Leeds where 92% of women questioned were in favour of routine enquiry by health professionals generally (Leeds Inter-Agency Project, 2005). It can be argued that health professionals, and particularly community midwives, are in an ideal position to ask women about domestic abuse. Not only do community midwives have access to a woman's body in a way that few other people do (and are therefore in a position to question any suspicious injuries), but they are also in a position to observe family interactions and build up a relationship with the woman that may lead to disclosure. Health directorates have recognised this and responded to it by including it in clinical practice recommendations.

The Royal College of Midwives, in Position Paper 19a (1999), state that 'the links between domestic abuse and adverse pregnancy outcomes suggest that midwives should assume a greater role in its detection and management'. One of the key recommendations of the Confidential Enquiry (Lewis, 2004) is that 'enquiries about violence should be routinely included when taking a social history at booking or at another opportune point in the antenatal period' and the *National Service Framework for Children, Young People and Maternity Services* (DH, 2004: 26) tells us that maternity service staff should be 'aware of the importance of domestic violence, competent in recognising the symptoms and presentations and able to make a sensitive enquiry and provide basic information and referral to local services'.

Routine enquiry about domestic violence during antenatal booking is still, however, infrequent (Foy et al., 2000). Even though midwives approve, in theory, of routine questioning about domestic abuse and broadly agree that it should form part of their responsibility (Price, 2004), practical and personal difficulties, including lack of time, staff shortages, and difficulty in obtaining sufficient privacy, were frequently cited as reasons why midwives do not ask the question (Leeds Inter-Agency Project, 2005). Fear of 'opening a can of worms' and lack of awareness and/or training about the issue are also cited by midwives as preventing them from asking the question. These concerns are being addressed with an action plan drawn up in response to the recommendations of the Domestic Abuse and Pregnancy Advisory Group (DH, 2005). These recommendations state that 'NHS maternity services should move to include a routine question as part of the social history taken during pregnancy, but this should be introduced at a measured pace with appropriate training' (DH, 2005: 111). Such training, along with other measures outlined in the action plan, should ensure that midwives will be able to ask pregnant women about domestic abuse confidently and safely.

Asking the question safely

Considerations of the safety of the pregnant woman and any existing children she may have are of utmost importance when raising the question of domestic abuse. It is vital to ensure that asking the question will not increase the level of danger or leave them feeling more vulnerable. Midwives need to consider how and where they are going to raise the subject and what they will need to do should disclosure follow.

As discussed earlier, the question of domestic abuse can be raised via selective screening of pregnant women exhibiting 'signs' or indicators of domestic abuse or by the routine enquiry of all pregnant women. Raising the question using selective screening will depend on when and where the 'signs' are identified. Clearly it would not be appropriate to raise the question when the partner or other family members are present because it is unlikely that a woman will disclose in front of others. Doing so may distress or embarrass her or even put her in further danger. It is advisable to make an appointment to see the woman alone wherever possible although this is easier said than done. Abusive partners are reluctant to leave their pregnant wives or girlfriends for fear that they may disclose what is happening. The DH (2005: 50) suggests that midwives may have to 'think creatively' about how they can access such women alone, such as 'when the woman is providing a urine sample or using the lavatory'. Even though this would give women a limited amount of time to talk and would not be the best environment for disclosure, it is better than not having the opportunity to ask the question at all.

Routine enquiry arguably makes it easier to ask the question. All women will be asked and this may take the stigma out of singling out certain women. Booking offers an ideal opportunity for midwives to raise the question as a matter of course when they are asking about other health and social factors. But it should be remembered that even when abuse is not suspected, women should not be asked the question in the presence of their partner or other family members, in fact it is good practice to ask pregnant women to attend the booking visit alone. This will not only give the midwife and the client the opportunity to talk, but could also reduce suspicion if the partner can be informed that this is a matter of procedure for all women. Ensuring that midwives ask the question to the woman while she is alone will also minimise any potential risk to the midwife, who must consider her own safety as well as the client's in this situation.

Before asking a direct question about domestic abuse, the reason for asking the question should be given. This puts the issue into context, i.e. it frames the question being asked and minimises the extent to which the woman may feel offended at being asked. The framing of the question will again depend upon the use of selective screening or routine enquiry. Framing questions using selective screening will revolve around the 'signs' that have caused concern and will inevitably need to be handled sensitively. If a woman has bruising on her abdomen, for example, the midwife will need to frame the question in terms of his/her concern about the bruises before asking any direct question about abuse.

On the other hand, routine enquiry gives the midwife the opportunity to frame the question according to policy and therefore offers a justification for asking a direct question about abuse. Some examples of framing the question for routine enquiry include:

- In addition to your health concerns, we are also asking all women about the possibility of intimate partner abuse within the home.
- As violence in the home is so common we now ask all women about it routinely.
- You may have seen our posters about domestic abuse outside. As part of our booking procedure we are asking all women about abuse in the home.

Standing Together Against Domestic Violence (2005: 5).

- 1 in 4 women in the UK will experience domestic abuse at some point in their lives. We also know that domestic abuse sometimes starts for the first time in pregnancy. That is why we are asking all pregnant women about this.

Bristol Pregnancy and Domestic Violence Programme (Baird et al., 2005: 25).

Once framed, a direct question can be asked. The application of a standardised question for all women during routine screening has been suggested (Garcia-Moreno, 2002); however, it is naïve to think that one question will suffice for all women, who naturally come from a wide range of cultural backgrounds. Variables such as age, sexuality, ability, etc. should be considered when choosing a question.

In Position Paper 19a, the RCM (1999) suggest that the following questions could be used:

- Is everything alright at home?
- How are you feeling?
- Are you getting the support you need at home?

These questions though are fairly vague and could be misconstrued so the RCM suggests some follow-up questions such as:

- I noticed a number of bruises/cuts/scratches/burn marks. How did they happen?
- Do you ever feel frightened of your partner?

Standing Together Against Domestic Violence (2005) offers similar suggestions for routine enquiry, including:

- Have you been physically hurt by your partner?
- Has your partner ever threatened to hurt you or someone you care about?
- Do you feel controlled and isolated by your partner? Does your partner belittle and insult you?

Such questions are much more direct and would need to be asked sensitively to reduce client discomfort and elicit disclosure (Hegarty and Taft, 2001). Mezey (1997) tells us that this type of direct questioning is necessary because it is rare for a woman experiencing domestic abuse to volunteer this information: most will only disclose if asked directly (though midwives should not assume that all women experiencing abuse will disclose upon questioning). For some women, feeling ashamed, harboring a belief that it is their problem or feeling that they should be able to manage it themselves are barriers to disclosure (Hegarty et al., 2005). These factors exist alongside the reality of a very intense fear of repercussions from their partner. For this reason it is advisable to repeat the question at intervals throughout the pregnancy, particularly where abuse is suspected. In addition, clinics should have posters, cards and pamphlets about domestic abuse on show and available for distribution. This will give the message that the clinic takes the problem seriously and may lead to women feeling more able to disclose, although it should be remembered that it may not be safe for a woman to take such information away with her in case the perpetrator finds it and assumes she has informed the midwife about the abuse. This would put the woman in an increased position of danger, as would sending any information relating to available support services through the post. The woman may be able to offer a safe address where information could be sent if she wishes.

Asking the question can, of course, lead to disclosure and it is important that midwives respond to disclosure appropriately and that they understand the limits of their role, which according to the DH (2005: 58) is to:

- help assess the risk to her and any children she has
- provide support and information to help the woman make a decision on what to do next
- encourage her to have a safety plan.

A flowchart by Devaney (2005), on behalf of the Leicester, Leicestershire and Rutland NHS Group, is a good example of the steps to follow after disclosure (Figure 11.1).

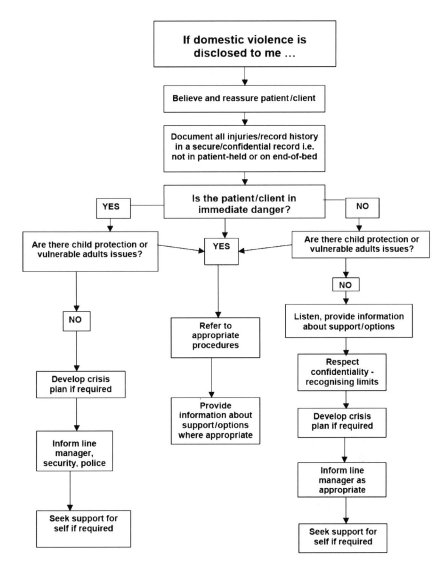

Figure 11.1 Model flowchart to follow when domestic violence is disclosed. Reproduced with permission from Carol Devaney.

According to Devaney (2005), the first and most essential thing that midwives should do is to believe and reassure the woman. This may be the first time that she has told anyone about what is happening to her, or she may have disclosed before and not been taken seriously. Research has highlighted the fact that women may disclose to between five and 12 different agencies before they get the help they need (Hester et al., 2000). Midwives should listen to what the woman has to say in a calm and non-judgemental manner. Professionals who react by exhibiting shock, alarm or distress may make the woman regret her decision to disclose.

Any disclosure of domestic abuse or injury relating to it should be documented as a matter of course in midwifery practice. The client's consent is not needed for such documentation as the recording of such information comes under the duty of care (NMC, 2002). However, it is important to explain to the woman why this is necessary and who will have access to the notes. It may help to explain that any recorded information could be used as part of any future legal case.

It is important that any record of disclosure can be accessed by all who care for the woman, but care has to be taken to maintain confidentiality and to ensure that the perpetrator does not find out about the disclosure. The DH (2005: 75) states that 'to ensure confidentiality, you should record domestic abuse separately from the main patient record and ensure that the record can only be accessed by those directly involved in the woman's care. *Domestic abuse should never be recorded in hand held notes, such as maternity notes'*.

Upon any disclosure of domestic abuse, midwives should assess the safety of the woman and any existing children by undertaking a risk assessment. Many trusts will have their own risk assessment procedures so it is important for midwives to familiarise themselves with these. However, as Devaney points out the first question to ask is 'Is the client in immediate danger?' (Devaney, 2005). If she is not and there are no child protection issues it may be appropriate to help the woman to develop a safety plan (Box 11.3), or simply to offer her the referral numbers of specialist agencies and organisations that can offer support and then monitor her progress through her pregnancy.

Box 11.3 What should be discussed when considering a safety plan?

- Current safety – is it safe go go home?
  - if NO discuss options and referrals
  - if YES consider:
    - safety strategies for inside and outside the home
    - safety plan to follow in an emergency
    - keeping children safe.

If the woman is in immediate danger or there are child protection issues, midwives will have a duty of care to share this information with appropriate agencies, even if the woman does not want her to. Child and/or vulnerable adult protection policies and procedures should be followed.

Ideally, the sharing of disclosed information should be done with consent and in many cases this can be obtained when a woman understands that it is for the good of her children or for her own safety. However, there will be cases where women flatly refuse and this can be distressing for both the woman and the midwife. In these situations it is important that midwives explain their duties and responsibilities, relating to disclosure, as sensitively and carefully as possible. Midwives are advised to access supervisory and managerial support in this difficult situation. A clear explanation of the process involved is required and this must include the woman as much as possible through extensive discussion relating to the rationale for the decisions made.

Confidentiality

To avoid confusion or any misunderstanding midwives should discuss confidentiality prior to asking the question about domestic abuse. They should inform and reassure the woman that any information disclosed will remain confidential unless there is concern for children, or for the woman's immediate safety, making it clear that if either such concerns became apparent, the midwife has a duty to share this information. It could be argued that informing the woman of this fact may prevent some women from disclosing, perhaps because of fear of police involvement or fear that they may have existing children removed from their care. It is not uncommon for perpetrators to threaten that this will happen if the abuse if discovered. Making the duty to disclose under these circumstances clear to women is extremely important because it will prevent them from feeling that they have been misled if the midwife does have to make the decision to share the disclosure. It is never possible to give an absolute promise of confidentiality.

All disclosed information about domestic abuse can legally be shared where necessary under the Crime and Disorder Act (Great Britain, 1998), Section 115, which makes it permissible to share information with another agency in situations where:

- the courts request information about a specific case
- there is significant risk of harm to the woman, her children or somebody else if the information is not shared.

The safety of the woman and her family should be considered before information is passed on. Midwives should be sure that sharing information will not put them at greater risk of violence. Guidance and support should be sought from senior colleagues before any information is shared. Further guidance on sharing information can be obtained from the Home Office publication *Safety and Justice: Sharing Personal Information in the Context of Domestic Violence* (Douglas et al., 2004). Midwives should also seek to familiarise themselves with their trust's confidentiality policies.

Legal issues

There are a number of specialist agencies and organisations to which midwives can refer women experiencing domestic abuse, either directly or by offering contact numbers (Box 11.4).

Box 11.4 Useful contact numbers

24-hour national domestic violence helplines:

- England
  0808 2000 247
- Wales
  080880 10 800
- Scotland
  0800 027 1234
- Northern Ireland
  0800 917 1414

Broken Rainbow
08452 604460
(Supports lesbian, gay, bisexual and transgender people who are experiencing domestic violence)

The most obvious agency in an emergency situation is the police. Historically, the police have not had the best reputation when it comes to dealing with domestic abuse, seeing it as a private matter between partners, but in recent years this has changed dramatically. All police officers now have comprehensive training in relation to domestic abuse and since recommendations were made by Her Majesty's Inspectorate of Constabulary in the early 1990s, most forces in England and Wales either have established specialist domestic violence units or employ specialist domestic violence officers. These specialist officers have had in-depth training and therefore understand the complex issues arising (Plotnikoff and Woolfson, 1998). Women who disclose domestic abuse can now expect to be taken seriously and treated sensitively by the police. Once the police are involved, the domestic abuse will become a criminal matter and midwives should ensure that their clients understand this because the police can proceed with a complaint regardless of the woman's wishes. Under recent legislation a woman cannot withdraw a complaint once it has been made (Great Britain, 2004a). The final decision about whether a case of domestic abuse will go to court will ultimately be up to the Crown Prosecution Service, but the important thing to remember is that the matter will be out of the woman's hands. The good news is that the Domestic Violence Crime and Victims Act (Great Britain, 2004b) has introduced new powers for the police and courts to deal with offenders, and improved support and protection for victims.

Historically there has not been a specific offence of 'domestic abuse' and this is not rectified under the Domestic Violence Crime and Victims Act (Great Britain, 2004b). Instead, it is dealt with under the Offences Against the Person Act (1861) and sections from other acts including:

- The Sexual Offences Act (1956)
- The Criminal Justice Act (1998)
- The Criminal Damage Act (1971)
- The Public Order Act (1986)
- The Criminal Justice and Public Order Act (1994)
- The Protection from Harassment Act (1997)
- The Domestic Violence Crime and Victims Bill (2004)

In addition to dealing with the offence, specialist domestic violence officers will also support women and will refer them on to a safe place to stay if deemed necessary. Such safe places are usually women's refuges, a network of accommodation across the UK that women can access via referrals from statutory agencies such as the police and health professionals (including midwives). Many safe houses can also be accessed through self-referral.

One option for a woman who does not want a criminal court case is to take civil action. There are six acts that apply in varying degrees to domestic violence in the civil jurisdiction:

- Part IV of the Family Law Act (1996)
- The Protection from Harassment Act (1997) (which also contains criminal sanctions)
- The Housing Act (1996)
- The Children Act (1989)
- The Adoption and Children Act (2002)
- The Domestic Violence, Crime and Victims Act (2004)

Under civil law a woman can apply to the court for orders such as a non-molestation injunction under the Family Law Act (1996). This restrains the perpetrator from approaching the woman, attacking her or from getting others to do so on their behalf. An occupation order is another option that regulates occupancy of the home.

It cannot be stressed enough that midwives should never attempt to give legal advice and should always refer women to the helpline or advise them to seek the help of a solicitor where they are indicating that they wish to take this route.

Refuges

Refuge accommodation offers a safe place for a woman and her children (if applicable) to stay but they can also offer information, support and advocacy, children's workers, counselling, resettlement services and much more depending on their financial situation. Refuges are not-for-profit organisations and therefore dependent on funding to provide services. Any woman and her children who are being abused can go into a refuge. There are specialist refuges that offer provision for disabled women and black and ethnic minority women (although it should never be assumed that black and minority ethnic women automatically want to go to a specialist refuge). Some refuges impose limitations on accepting women with mental health problems or with alcohol or drug dependency. This is because they have to consider the safety of other women and children resident in the refuge at all times. Also, for this reason, some refuges have an age limit on accepting male children of women. This is often set at 14 years of age but this proviso can be older or younger. It is vital for midwives to check these anomalies with the refuge provider before referring a woman there. A useful tool for midwives and indeed all practitioners is the *Gold Book* published by Women's Aid, which contains annually updated details of refuge providers and their admissions policies.

There are a number of other services that midwives could offer information about or refer women to according to their needs. These needs may include practical matters and referrals could be made to such organisations as the Benefits Agency, Housing or Citizens Advice, or more personal needs relating to health such as alcohol and drug dependency, mental health, sexual health, etc. The client may also have social and cultural needs such as matters relating to ethnicity and sexuality and may need help or advice from related specialist services. Many women can have a variety of complex and overlapping needs requiring a number of services and this can be daunting for both the woman and the midwife. With this in mind, it is recommended that midwives use national or local domestic abuse helplines for advice and that they offer the helpline number to the client in non-emergency situations. These helplines have been set up specifically to assist with the complex needs of women experiencing domestic abuse. They can offer a listening ear and signposts to information, practical and legal advice, outreach services and referrals to refuges. All helpline workers are trained to a high standard on the many issues surrounding domestic abuse and this service should be utilised in order to ensure that the women get the help they need and that midwives do not become engulfed with dealing with this difficult situation. Community midwives should not be expected to act as counsellors, nor should they be expected to solve the situation. Their role should be to respond effectively by listening, assessing safety, documenting the disclosure and making referrals where necessary and appropriate. This should hopefully reassure midwives who may fear that they would be expected to deal with the issue all by themselves and as a result have not asked the all-important question.

Referring to appropriate agencies/organisations will also ensure that women get the correct information. Midwives cannot be expected to be able to answer all the questions a woman may have in relation to the abuse and one of the most complex questions may relate to what the woman can do legally without getting the police involved.

Women from black and other ethnic minority backgrounds

It is important to note in this chapter that domestic abuse can be directed toward any woman regardless of class, (dis)ability, sexuality, age and ethnicity and midwives should recognise this fact. However, it is important to pay particular consideration to domestic abuse perpetrated against women from black and other minority ethnic backgrounds. This is not because they are more likely to become victims, but because we live in a multi-cultural society. The 2001 Census revealed that the UK today is more culturally diverse than ever before (UK Census, 2001) and, as a result, midwives will have clients from a wide variety of cultural backgrounds. In addition, the Women's Aid Federation of England tell us that 'the form the abuse takes may vary; in some communities, for example, domestic violence may be perpetrated by extended family members, or it may include forced marriage, or female genital mutilation. Women from black or minority ethnic communities may also be more isolated, or may have to overcome religious and cultural pressures, and they may be afraid of bringing shame onto their "family honour"' (Women's Aid, 2006; Case study 11.1).

Case study 11.1

Rukhsana Naz, a 19-year-old in the advanced stages of pregnancy, was strangled in 1998 by her mother and her 22-year-old brother, Shazad, after she had shamed them by conceiving out of wedlock.

When her younger brother chanced upon them, his mother said, 'Be strong, son' as she forced him to help dispose of Rukhsana's body.

(Alam, 2004)

There are many cultural and religious stereotypes relating to black and other ethnic minority women. This may lead to midwives being unsure about how to respond, or being unwilling to respond to situations where they think that abuse may be taking place, for fear of challenging what they see as cultural traditions and perhaps for fear of appearing to be racist. Equally, women may not seek help because they anticipate encountering a racist response. In addition, there may be language barriers for those women who do not speak any English and who rely entirely on a partner or another family member to communicate. Midwives should never accept that what the partner or family member is translating to them is correct but should seek an independent interpreter.

Domestic abuse is never acceptable for any woman. Regardless of race and ethnicity, midwives should respond to suspected abuse or use routine enquiry in the same way as they would for any other woman, using the same procedures and protocol. When raising the question, midwives should ensure that they do so when they are alone with the woman (using an interpreter where necessary) and should do so sensitively, responding to disclosure in exactly the same way as they would with any other woman; documenting the interaction and using appropriate referral services where applicable.

There are a number of specialist services for women from black and ethnic minorities, and women may be in particular need of these if they have insecure immigration status (Box 11.5).

Box 11.5 Useful numbers

Southall Black Sisters
020 8571 9595

Asylum Aid
020 7247 8741

Multikulti: Provides information in a number of community languages (as well as English) on issues such as immigration, claiming asylum, health, housing, welfare benefits and employment. Website: www.multikulti.org.uk

Immigration Advisory Service
0207 378 9191
www.iasuk.org

Panahghar: Help for Asian women experiencing domestic abuse
01203 228952

Chinese Information and Advice Centre
020 7692 3697

Current immigration rules state that women coming to this country to join a partner who is already living here have to complete a 2-year probationary period during which time they must live with their partner before they can make an application for indefinite leave to remain in the UK. If women leave their partners before the 2-year probationary period is completed they will have no recourse to public funds. This means they will not be able to claim state benefits and this will, of course, make it much more difficult for them to leave the abuser.

Understanding that she has insecure immigration status may make the woman more reluctant to disclose the abuse for fear of being deported, so it is paramount that midwives reassure such women about the fact that 'regardless of immigration status they are entitled to protection and that the abuser is subject to the same sanctions as other abusers regardless of his immigration status' (Women's Aid, 2006). Such women must be reassured that if they can prove that they are experiencing domestic abuse, they can apply for indefinite leave to remain in the UK.

It is important that midwives do not try to advise black and other ethnic minority women about their immigration status or financial rights. This must be the role of expert legal representatives and referral must be made to appropriate agencies with the woman's consent where possible, but it is appropriate to do this without consent if the midwife feels that the woman is in immediate danger.

Midwives should also never automatically refer women to agencies/organisations specifically for black and other ethnic minority women. Such women may prefer to use general services as they think it will be easier for their partners to trace them through specialist services and may fear being judged by workers from the same cultural background. Again, midwives may want to elicit the advice of workers staffing national or local domestic abuse helplines.

Before making any referrals whatsoever concerning any woman, regardless of ethnicity, age, sexuality, (dis)ability, etc., midwives should familiarise themselves with the policy and practice guidelines of their Trust and if in doubt should seek the advice of senior colleagues.

Inter-agency working

The complexity of domestic abuse and the many agencies that may need to be involved, combined with the need at times to share information, means that inter-agency working is both necessary and important for the safety of the woman and any children she may have and for effective service provision. The Home Office issued a circular encouraging the inter-agency coordination of domestic violence in 1995, on behalf of the Inter-Departmental Group on Domestic Violence (Home Office, 1995). Inter-agency responses to domestic abuse usually take the form of domestic abuse forums, bringing all relevant statutory and voluntary sector agencies together (Malos, 1998). There are currently over 200 domestic abuse forums across the UK (Women's Aid, 2006). Forums typically include representation from the police, local refuges, social services, housing departments, probation and voluntary sector agencies. Malos (1998) has stated that representation by health services has frequently been absent, although their greater involvement would be widely welcomed. Since then, this has changed a great deal with more and more health providers getting involved with forums and with addressing domestic abuse generally in an attempt to increase the safety of abused women and children. PCTs in England became 'responsible authorities under the Crime and Disorder Act 1998, amended by the Police Reform Act 2002, on 30th April 2004' (DH/Home Office, 2004). This means that PCTs now have a statutory duty to work in partnership with other agencies to reduce crime. This includes working to reduce domestic abuse and midwives play a pivotal role in this move through routine enquiry.

Summary

Routine enquiry for domestic abuse has yet to be incorporated into everyday midwifery practice in every NHS Trust. Yet domestic abuse is a problem far more prevalent than gestational diabetes, pre-eclampsia or unexplained stillbirth – potential problems that midwives routinely screen for as a matter of course (Wright, 2003), but there are moves under way to address this. The DH (2000) has endorsed routine antenatal enquiry for domestic violence and they have been followed by the Royal College of Obstetricians and Gynaecologists, the RCM and NICE. In 2000, the DH also awarded The Women's Aid Federation of England £85 540 over 3 years to raise awareness of domestic abuse amongst health professionals and to introduce a resource manual to NHS staff. This manual was published in 2000 and updated in 2005 (Women's Aid, 2006).

The manual stresses the importance of training staff about domestic abuse as a precursor to effective screening, highlighting the fact that implementing screening interventions without sufficient training, resources and support for midwives could be dangerous for both women and midwives. A study in Bristol (Price, 2004) where 79 midwives were trained in routine screening for domestic abuse and related issues, concluded that the training was 'positively received by participants, particularly in relation to an increased awareness of and confidence in dealing with the issue and that the training had an impact on the level of disclosure facilitated by midwives'.

I believe that training midwives about domestic abuse is essential in order to sustain routine enquiry and to ensure that midwives are aware of how to respond to disclosure in a way that will ensure the safety of the woman and any children she has. Training should not only be about women and child protection but also about the safety of the midwives asking the question. Community midwives in particular, who go into the homes of clients and often work alone, may be put in a dangerous position if they are not trained in asking about domestic abuse safely. Any domestic abuse training programme should include safety advice relating to lone working, undertaking home visits and responding to aggression. The RCM does offer direction on this in Position Paper no. 12 *Safety for Midwives Working in the Community* (RCM, 1996).

Finally, raising the question of domestic abuse with women should not be undertaken by midwives without policies and procedures being firmly in place. As Garcia-Moreno tells us 'well motivated changes may have harmful outcomes' (cited in Hegarty et al., 2005). Robotham (2000) comments that midwives have frequently been the identifiers of abuse but are often hampered in their efforts to deal with it, as they are unsure who to turn to for advice. Providing supervision for midwives is imperative for routine enquiry to work, as is the recognition that with the majority of midwives being women there is a high probability that many will be survivors of domestic abuse themselves, or may even presently be in an abusive relationship. Provision must be made, therefore, for these women to be supported both in terms of their own experiences and in terms of giving them the confidence to raise the question of domestic abuse with their clients.

PCTs are responding to the need for routine screening. Many have guidelines in place and others are implementing strategies as this chapter goes to press. Such screening has been shown to increase the identification of domestic abuse (Price, 2004) and is, in my opinion, a necessary and potentially life-saving move. If implemented nationally it will not only save lives but will also reduce the colossal £1.4 billion that Sylvia Walby (Walby and Allen, 2004) calculated domestic abuse costs the NHS every year in her government report. What more evidence or justification do we need?

🔑 Key points

When undertaking routine enquiry, remember to use your RADAR!

Routine enquiry	Never implement routine enquiry without training and support
Ask to be alone	Never ask a client about domestic abuse in the presence of her partner, other family members or friends
Document after Disclosure	Respond non-judgementally to disclosure and document it according to your trust's policy on recording information and confidentiality
Assess safety	Always be aware of the safety of the client, any children she may have and your own safety. Help client draw up a safety plan if necessary
Refer to specialist agencies	Accept the boundaries of your role – use specialist agencies/organisations where necessary

RADAR model adapted from the American Medical Association (1992).

References

Alam, F. (2004) Take the honour out of killing. *The Guardian,* Tuesday July 6th.

American Medical Association (1992) *Diagnostic and Treatment Guidelines on Domestic Violence.* American Medical Association, Chicago, IL.

Bacchus, L., Mezey, G. and Bewly, S. (2002) Women's perceptions and experiences of routine enquiry for domestic violence in a maternity service. *International Journal of Obstetrics and Gynaecology,* **109**, 9–16

Baird, K., Price, S. and Salmon, D. (2005) *Bristol Pregnancy and Domestic Violence Programme: Training Manual.* University of the West of England, Bristol.

DH (2000) *Domestic Violence: A Resource Manual for Health Professionals,* Department of Health, London.

DH (2004) *National Service Framework for Children, Young People and Maternity Services: Part 11 Maternity Standard.* Gateway ref. 3779, Department of Health, London.

DH (2005) *Responding to Domestic Abuse: A Handbook for Health Professionals.* The Stationery Office, London.

DH/Home Office (2004) *Guidance for Partnerships and Primary Care Trusts.* Department of Health/Home Office, London.

Devaney, C. (2005) *Model Flowchart for When Domestic Violence is Disclosed.* Leicestershire and Rutland NHS Group, Leicester.

Douglas, N., et al. (2004) *Safety and Justice: Sharing Personal Information in the Context of Domestic Violence: An Overview.* Home Office report No. 30.

Flood-Page, C. and Taylor, M.J. (eds) (2003) *Crime in England and Wales 2001/2002: Supplementary Volume*. Home Office, London. Available at http://www.homeoffice.gov.uk/rds/pdfs2/hosb103.pdf/

Foy, R., Nelson, F., Penney, G. and McIlwaine, G. (2000) Antenatal detection of domestic violence. *The Lancet*, **355** (9218), 1915.

Garcia-Moreno, C. (2002) Dilemmas and opportunities for an appropriate health service response to violence against women. *The Lancet*, **359** (9316), 1509–1514.

Great Britain (1998) *Crime and Disorder Act 1998 (c37)*, HMSO, London.

Great Britain (2004a) *Domestic Violence Crime and Justice Bill 2004*, HMSO, London.

Great Britain (2004b) *Domestic Violence Crime and Victims Act 2004 (c28)*, HMSO, London.

Hegarty, K. and Taft, A. (2001) Overcoming the barriers to disclosure and inquiry of partner abuse for women attending general practice. *Australian and New Zealand Journal of Public Health*, **25** (4), 433–438.

Hegarty, K., Feder, G. and Ramsay, J. (2005) Identification of intimate partner abuse in health care settings: Should health professionals be screening? In *Intimate Partner Abuse and Health Professionals: New Approaches to Domestic Violence* (eds G. Roberts et al.). Elsevier Health Sciences, Edinburgh.

Hester, M., Pearson, C. and Harwin, N. (2000) *Making an Impact: Children and Domestic Violence: A Reader*. Jessica Kingsley, London.

Home Office (1995) *Inter-Agency Co-Ordination to Tackle Domestic Violence*. Home Office Inter-Agency Circular, London.

Kershaw, C., Chivite-Matthews, N., Thomas, C. and Aust, R. (2001) *The 2001 British Crime Survey: First Results, England and Wales*. The Home Office, London.

Leeds Inter-Agency Project (2005) *Health and Social Care Project Report: Promoting Good Practice in Health Service Responses to Women and Children Experiencing Domestic Violence*. LIAP, Leeds.

Lewis, G. (ed.) (2001) *Why Mothers Die: Report from the Confidential Enquiries into Maternal Deaths in the UK 1997-9*. RCOG, London.

Lewis, G. (ed.) (2004) *Why Mothers Die 2000–2002 – Report on Confidential Enquiries into Maternal Deaths in the United Kingdom*. RCOG, London.

Malos, E. (1998) *Domestic Violence: Action for Change*, 2nd edn, New Clarion Press, Cheltenham.

McWilliams, M. and McKinnon, M. (1993) *Bringing it out in the Open: Domestic Violence in Northern Ireland*. HMSO, Belfast.

Mezey, G. (1997) *Domestic violence in pregnancy*. In *Violence Against Women* (eds. S. Bewley, J. Friend, G. Mezey). RCOG, London.

Mezey, G., et al. (2003) Midwives' perceptions and experiences of routine enquiry for domestic violence. *British Journal of Obstetrics and Gynaecology*, **110**, 744–752.

Mooney, J. (1993) *The Hidden Figure: Domestic Violence in North London*. Islington Police and Crime Prevention Unit, London.

Newberger, Eli, H., et al. (1992) Abuse of pregnant women and adverse birth outcome. *Journal of the American Medical Association*, **267** (17), 2370–2372.

NMC (2002) *Guidelines for Records and Record Keeping*. Nursing and Midwifery Council, London.

Plotnikoff, J. and Woolfson, R. (1998) *Policing Domestic Violence: Effective Organisational Structures*. Police Research Series, Paper 100, Home Office, London.

Price, S. (2004) Routine questioning about domestic violence in maternity settings. *Midwives*, **7**, 4 April.

Ramsay, J., Richardson, J., Carter, Y.H., Davidson, L.L. and Feder, G. (2002) Should health professionals screen women for domestic violence? *British Medical Journal*, **325**, 314–318.

Robotham, M. (2000) You can't beat togetherness. *Nursing Times*, **96** (12), 30–31.

RCM (1996) *Safety for Midwives Working in the Community: Position Paper 12*. Royal College of Midwives, London.

RCM (1999) *Domestic Abuse in Pregnancy: Position Paper 19a*. Royal College of Midwives, London.

Standing Together against Domestic Violence: Intimate Partner Violence Screening Tool (2005) www.standingtogether.org.uk (accessed June 2006).

Taket, A., Nurse, J., Smith, K., Watson, J. and Shakespeare, J. (2003) Routinely asking women about domestic violence in health settings. *British Medical Journal*, **327**, 673–676.

UK Census (2001) cited by Office of National Statistics in Ethnicity and Identity. http://www.statistics.gov.uk/focuson/ethnicity (accessed June 2006).

Viner, K. (2005) A year of killing. *The Guardian*, Saturday December 10th.

Walby, S. and Allen, J. (2004) *Domestic Violence, Sexual Assault and Stalking: Findings from the British Crime Survey*. Home Office Development and Statistics Directorate: Research Study 276, London.

Waalen, J., Goodwin, M.M., Spitz, A.M., Petersen, R. and Saltzman, L.E. (2000) Screening for intimate partner violence by health care providers: barriers and interventions. *Journal of Preventive Medicine*, **19**, 230–237.

Women's Aid (2006) Women from Black and minority ethnic communities. In *The Survivors Handbook*. Women's Aid Federation of England. www.womensaid.org.uk (accessed June 2006).

WHO (2000) *Violence against women; Fact sheet 239*. World Health Organization, Geneva.

Wright, L. (2003) Asking about domestic violence. *British Journal of Midwifery*, **11** (4), 199–202.

Suggested further reading

Aston, G. (2004) The silence of domestic violence in pregnancy during women's encounters with healthcare professionals. *Midwives*, **7**, 4.

Bacchus, L. (2004) Domestic violence and health. *Midwives*, **7**, 4.

Feder, G., Hutson, M., Ramsay, J. and Taket, A. (2006) Expectations and experiences of women experiencing intimate partner violence when they encounter health care professionals: A meta-analysis of qualitative studies. *Archives of Internal Medicine*, **166**, 22–37.

Fogarty, C. (2002) Communication with patients about intimate partner violence: Screening and interviewing approaches. *Family Medicine*, **34** (5), 369–375.

Taket, A. (2004) Tackling domestic violence: The role of health professionals. Home Office Development and Practice Report 32. Home Office, London. Available at http://www.homeoffice.gov.uk/rds/pdfs04/dpr32.pdf.

12

Pelvic girdle pain (formerly known as symphysis pubis dysfunction)

Dianne Garland

'The pain was like an aching in my pubic bone and groin area, which then became a burning feeling in my groin and a "clicking" feeling when I walked. Nobody ever gave a name to the pain, both the midwives and doctors said it was part of being pregnant and that it was normal. However, my GP was very understanding as she knew I couldn't work, but again could not give it a name. After my delivery I had hydrocortisone injections in my groin and these have helped. It's now several years later and I believe that midwives are more helpful and understanding of the condition.'
'K'– a mother with pelvic girdle pain

Recent European Commission guidelines (Vleeming et al., 2004) indicate that it is time to reconsider the use of the term 'symphysis pubis dysfunction' (SPD). To achieve consistency, it should now be referred to as 'pelvic girdle pain' (PGP). This terminology is much more appropriate because it indicates the involvement of the whole pelvis and not just the symphysis pubis.

Various authors have attempted to identify the incidence of PGP and Andrew (2005) states that 20% of pregnant women have this condition, with 5% experiencing serious problems. Wellock (Wellock et al., 2005) writes that she believes as many as 1 in 27 to 1 in 36 women could be affected. Other authors quote figures of 1 in 250, or some 3000 women per year in the UK.

During my midwifery training in 1982, I am positive that no-one ever mentioned PGP. However, it must be recognised that awareness of the condition was generally non-existent at that time and that women's symptoms were generally put down to the physiological changes of pregnancy. I don't think that my opinion is unique. Having spoken to many midwives who trained at the same time, they agree that we had little input into this condition that manifests itself acutely and/or chronically to cause significant physical and psychological distress.

Subsequently, understanding of PGP has grown enormously. PGP has such a profound effect on both the woman and her family that they often need support in accessing alternative therapies when conventional therapy has failed. It is a real challenge for any midwife to help a woman redesign her lifestyle realistically. Women with PGP need the support of a community midwife to cope with the condition in pregnancy from day to day and to achieve a satisfying birth. The global objectives of this chapter are to provide insights from a practising midwife's perspective and to offer practical advice. This should enable the reader to offer effective support for women with this condition.

The pelvic girdle is made up of three large bones, comprising the sacrum (or base of the spine) and two ilea. These isometric bones are commonly known as the hip bones and meet to form the joint at the front of the pelvis known as the symphysis pubis. Posteriorly, they are attached to the sacrum by the sacroiliac joints (Figure 12.1).

Early studies have tended to focus on the symphysis pubis in an attempt to differentiate between PGP and back problems in pregnancy. There is evidence to suggest that asymmetric laxity of the sacroiliac joints may be responsible for some of the pain and dysfunction of PGP (Franke, 2003). The condition was recognised as early as the time of Hippocrates and 'joint loosening' of the pelvis was described in the literature as early as 1839. During the latter part of the 20th century, very little was documented to aid recognition and improve

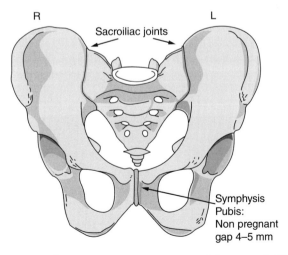

Figure 12.1 Normal presentation. © Lippincott, Williams and Wilkins LifeART Collection.

awareness of PGP until the formation of the British SPD support group in 1995.

Recognising and diagnosing pelvic girdle pain

The normal non-pregnant physiological gap between the symphysis pubis is 4 mm. When the degree of separation of the symphysis pubis measures between 4 and 10 mm it is defined as SPD, whilst a gap greater than 10 mm is called diastasis symphysis pubis (Figure 12.2). For the majority of women these terms are irrelevant since the amount of pain experienced may not be in relation to the size of the gap.

Aetiology

There have been various theories and thoughts regarding the aetiology of PGP. These have included familial, metabolic, biochemical, anatomical and even geographical; however, no author has been able to identify one single factor and the condition is thought to be multi-factorial. There is some suggestion that mothers who have experienced an early menarche may be more susceptible (Leadbetter et al., 2004). Leadbetter et al. also suggest that there is a familial tendency in prevalence between mothers, daughters or sisters, a relationship with calcium levels, links to previous anatomical problems and a history of any medical illness or accident involving the mother's back, hips, neck or pelvic areas. All are thought to predispose women to PGP in pregnancy (Case study 12.1).

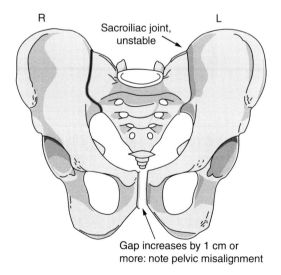

Figure 12.2   Diastasis symphysis pubis. © Lippincott, Williams and Wilkins LifeART Collection.

Case study 12.1 Hollingworth and Hawley's (1994) case

Hollingworth and Hawley report the case of a 22-year-old Asian woman in her first pregnancy who developed disabling pelvic girdle pain from 26 weeks. A diagnosis of sacroiliac and symphysis pubis joint pain was made and she was managed with simple analgesics, physiotherapy and eventually bed rest. There were no risk factors in her past medical history and the woman had lived in Britain all her life.

Blood tests revealed severe vitamin D deficiency. Lumbar spine and pelvic X-rays identified osteopenic bones with pseudo fractures, most notably in the left suprapubic ramus. A bone biopsy showed excessive osteoid formation, consistent with osteomalacia. The mother was given a stat dose of 100 000 international units of calciferol orally and Sandocal 1 g daily, three calcium and vitamin D tablets per day, and one multivitamin tablet per day. Within 2 weeks her vitamin D and parathyroid hormone levels were improving. Within 2 months there was a clear improvement in her walking and pain was reduced. Treatment was continued for a further 3 months.

The authors conclude that pelvic girdle pain presenting in pregnancy in Asian women should prompt consideration of osteomalacia as a possible underlying cause.

Wellock (2002) identifies several biomechanical influences. These include the effects of relaxin, oestrogen and progesterone. However, once again, there appears to be no conclusive evidence relating to one individual factor and this theory has been questioned by other authors (Kristiansson et al., 1996).

Interestingly, there appears to be a higher recorded prevalence of PGP in Northern Europe (Vangen et al., 1999). This might be due to a heightened awareness and reporting of the condition, achieved through good communication between midwives and pregnant women and the work of consumer support groups that raise awareness of PGP via the media and the internet.

Diagnosis

PGP is often misdiagnosed due to a lack of knowledge, inadequate clinical examination or mixed signs and symptoms. Women have been quoted as being misdiagnosed with urinary tract infections, round ligament pain, nerve compression, bone infections and even pre-term labour. It is no wonder that women feel frustrated and health professionals uncertain. Ostgaard et al. (1994) differentiated between PGP and sciatica. PGP has a less specific nerve root syndrome distribution and rarely radiates down to the ankle or the foot. The pain does not include muscle weakness or sensory impairment, and reflexes are unchanged.

The active straight leg raise test (ASLR) is one of the tests recommended by the European Commission (Vleeming et al., 2004). The woman lies in a supine position with straight legs and the feet positioned 20 cm apart. The assessor (often a physiotherapist) then asks the woman to raise each leg individually, one after the other, until it is 20 cm above the couch. During the ASLR it is important to avoid bending the knees. Mens et al. (2001) describe how the woman should then be asked to score their impairment on a 6-point scale ranging from 'not difficult at all' (0) to 'unable to do' (5). The scores for the right and left sides are added together to arrive at a sum total ranging from 0 to 10 (Box 12.1).

Box 12.1 Related research

Albert et al. (2000) attempted to evaluate methods of assessing pelvic pain in pregnancy through scrutiny of 15 clinical tests. They concluded that a reliable test is yet to be developed and that standardisation and skilled examination are needed to improve diagnosis. On a practical level this does show how difficult it is to assess, test and diagnose PGP.

There are limited indications for the use of conventional radiography in the diagnosis of PGP, due to its poor sensitivity, but magnetic resonance imaging scanning may help to diagnose the problem definitively in severe cases.

Good practice relating to the evaluation of PGP includes recording a pain history with particular attention to pain caused through prolonged periods of standing and/or sitting. In order to differentiate diagnoses and ensure that the pain is related to the pelvic girdle it is important to locate the site of the pain accurately. Vleeming et al. (2004) suggest that asking the patient to shade in the area affected on a pain location diagram is more reliable than merely asking them to point to the exact location (Box 12.2).

Box 12.2 Practice point

In pregnant women with PGP the range of hip movements will be limited by pain and there will be an inability to tolerate the palpation of the symphysis pubis, which may be very obvious during routine antenatal check-ups. Health professionals must always take great care during abdominal palpation and with the use of Pawlik's grip in particular.

Physical signs and symptoms

The clinical picture may have a sudden or chronic onset, with a variety of symptoms, some classical and others more diverse. Classic symptoms are pain over the symphysis pubis, which is very painful to touch, or pain in the lower abdomen that radiates down the woman's inner thighs. The latter is often described as a shooting type of pain.

Pain may be most noticeable during the daily activities of normal life. The nature of the pain can change and may increase or be exacerbated with walking, lifting one leg whilst going up or down stairs, getting into bed, getting into a bath, turning over in bed or rising from a deep chair. This classical symptom is usually relieved by resting. Women often report the distressing experience of a clicking, snapping or grinding sensation, which can be heard or felt within the symphysis pubis. Midwives can perform a clinical examination if women report these distressing signs and symptoms, but it might initially be more appropriate to ask the woman if she is experiencing any pain during daily activity.

On examination the mother may be tender over the symphysis pubis or sacroiliac joints. There could also be a palpable pubic gap or even suprapubic oedema. As the woman enters the room for a routine appointment the midwife may observe that she has a classic waddling gait. Less classic symptoms are dysuria or, occasionally, difficulty in voiding.

Psychosocial issues

It is commonly acknowledged that PGP has a profound psychological impact on both the woman and her family. It is not uncommon to hear women saying that 'No-one believes me' and, even worse, 'No-one cares'. The psychological effects for women may present as depression, resentment, anger, lack of self-esteem and lack of confidence.

Family relationships are undoubtedly altered with women describing changes affecting the dynamics of their marriage, including their sex life (Wellock, 2002). Another significant impact of PGP is the effect on social life. Not being able to go out because of restricted mobility, or embarrassment at using crutches, has an isolating effect that can be linked to depression (Shepherd, 2005). The status of working women can also alter as anecdotal reports indicate that not all employers are sympathetic to immobile pregnant women using crutches, frequent professional visits, hospital admissions or home care. The Health and Safety Executive (HSE, 2007) offers comprehensive advice to employers whose employees are living with musculoskeletal disorders in general. They suggest clear strategies to support employees and one of these strategies is to agree a return to work plan. This might include working on different tasks, working shorter hours, adapting the work environment and even assisting with transport. The HSE emphasises that the employee should not be pressurised to return to work. Such a plan could make the difference between returning to work or subsequent unemployment and the associated potential for financial hardship.

Existing young children can encounter difficulties adjusting to the changes that PGP brings for their mother. It is hard to explain to a toddler the reasons why mummy can no longer play with them. This has the potential to significantly undermine a woman's confidence in her parenting abilities. A study by Wellock et al. (2005) identifies four key areas of concern for women living with PGP, and their carers, that reiterate the difficulties associated with the condition:

- Women's perceptions of pain are described with emotive words (such as raw, throbbing, stabbing, sharp, shocking) that illustrate an extremely difficult experience.
- Distressing audible crunching, cracking, clunking and clicking sounds are heard by the woman and sometimes her partner.
- Negative effects upon the role of the woman within the family unit are clear – she can't pick up her toddler; her abilities as a 'domestic goddess' are greatly compromised.
- Interactions with health professionals are difficult – GP are quoted as offering negative plaudits such as 'grin and bear it' and the reactions attributed to midwives are mixed.

These issues highlight the urgent need for midwives to respond to the needs of women. Maintaining a positive mental attitude is possible if the midwife can facilitate connection with peer groups such as the British DSP support group (www.spd-uk.org) or the Pelvic Partnership (www.pelvicpartnership.org.uk). Appropriate literature and detailed planning for the birth of the baby can give the woman many positive aspects to focus on.

Management

Midwives are constantly working to provide woman-centred care but may feel daunted at the prospect of making a difference to women who have PGP. There is a lot that can be done to support a woman with this problem and it is important to emphasise the positive interventions that exist. Although it sounds obvious, the first measure is actually to recognise PGP as early as possible.

Antenatal care

During pregnancy, effective support from the community midwife needs to encompass psychosocial and physical needs. If midwives are aware of the following practical tips they can make realistic suggestions that can improve the woman's quality of life.

- *Encourage the woman to listen to her body*. She needs to identify the activities that cause discomfort and then try to avoid, stop or reduce the activity, i.e. prolonged standing, excessive walking, exercise. Although swimming breast stroke is not thought to be good, because the unnatural leg action could place extra strain on the pelvic girdle, it does depend on the individual woman.

- *Avoid heavy lifting whenever possible.* If a toddler has to be lifted it is possible to use persuasion to get him or her to climb on a stool or chair first.
- *Advise the woman to rest* in the position that is most comfortable for her (sitting or lying) to take the weight off her pelvis. It might also be possible to sit down to undertake normal daily activities like ironing and cooking. Occupational therapists can assess the woman's needs and provide aids such as bath seats and perching stools for ironing or showering.
- *Increasing the height of a sofa or armchair* with extra cushions is a simple measure that will make it easier for the woman to get up from the chair.
- *Consider the use of aids* such as a claw to pick up objects and a wheelchair when shopping may also help. It is important that the woman feels comfortable with these aids and does not feel embarrassed.
- *Avoid straddling movements*, especially when getting in or out of the car, chairs or bed. When getting out of bed, keep both legs together, bend and keep the knees together and avoid twisting movements. Walking up stairs is difficult and it may be wise to move sideways like a crab, or on your bottom.
- *Plan the day's activities.* This is a useful strategy that can minimise the number of times a woman has to go up and down stairs. Have the telephone and remote controls for the television to hand to avoid extra movement.
- *Recommend referral to a specialist physiotherapist.* They will be able to provide trochanteric belts or double tubigrip if pain is severe. Pelvic supports, like a trochanteric belt or tubigrip, and elbow crutches may help because they take the weight off the pelvis. A physiotherapist will also be able to provide advice on back care, reduction and management of joint dysfunction and correction of muscle imbalance (ACPWH, 1996; Box 12.3).

Box 12.3 Related research

A randomised clinical trial (Depledge et al., 2005) was designed to compare muscle strengthening exercises and advice regarding daily activities against rigid or non-rigid pelvic support belts.

Various measurement tools were utilised, including Roland–Morris questionnaire scoring, Patient Specific Functional Scale scoring and average/worst pain scores. All study groups showed significant improvement in function over time but no difference between the groups. Belts made no difference but they did help women to use their muscles and provide stability to the pelvis.

Maintaining mobility is a priority. It is well documented that pregnant women are at risk of thromboembolism with prolonged bed rest. If a woman with PGP is admitted to hospital antenatally, anti-embolism stockings and low molecular weight heparin may be used prophylactically to reduce maternal morbidity and mortality (Lewis, 2001).

Mobility will be maximised if pain is controlled. Refer women to their GP to request analgesia and/or anti-inflammatory drugs to be prescribed from 16 weeks. Bear in mind that codeine-based analgesics taken over time can lead to constipation so the amount and type of analgesia need to be reviewed regularly. It might be necessary to refer onwards to a specialist pain clinic if GP-prescribed analgesia or anti-inflammatory drugs do not control pain adequately.

Acupuncture, chiropractic, osteopathy and aromatherapy may have beneficial effects for some individuals (Wedenberg et al., 2000) and some women will want to use complementary therapies during the antenatal period. The European Commission (Vleeming et al., 2004) recommends that acupuncture should be considered in pregnancy and a recent randomised single-blind study by Elden et al. (2005) concluded that acupuncture and stabilising exercises are beneficial in conjunction with standard treatments for the management of PGP during pregnancy. Interestingly, in this small study of 386 women acupuncture was actually found to be superior to stabilising exercises in attenuating PGP.

It is vital that consumers are aware of the professional background of any complementary therapist and his or her qualifications. It would also be a sensible idea to ask the therapist about other cases of PGP that they have treated, and their outcomes (Andrew, 2005). If a pregnant woman is using complementary therapies it may also be worth considering the use of transcutaneous nerve stimulation (TENS). A physiotherapist must supervise the use of TENS during pregnancy. Midwives are only covered in its use for women in labour after 37 weeks' gestation.

PGP is now acknowledged as a reality for many women in pregnancy but the pain will not always resolve quickly after the birth of the baby. Referral to other agencies may be appropriate, i.e. social services and health visitors, who can help the family to plan for the postnatal period.

Self-help groups and local or national support groups should be known to midwives, who can help by putting women in touch with others who have PGP. Peer support from those who can identify with the experience is invaluable in reducing feelings of isolation. Friends and family should naturally be involved too. It is very important that all members of the woman's family are aware of the restrictions that PGP places upon her, and the best ways to support her both physically and psychologically.

Pre-planning options for labour and birth are important for any woman. However, with PGP, a birth plan not only helps to negotiate what is and is not possible for her; but it also offers the midwives caring for her in labour (who may not know the woman) clear information to ensure effective care provision and support. A good time to formulate a birth plan is round about 36 weeks. By this time the woman will have a good idea of her own mobility and restrictions. The plan should incorporate aspects of care relating to positions for labour, analgesia and birth modes. A sample birth plan can be found on the National Childbirth Trust (NCT) website.

Measuring the pain-free gap should be undertaken by the midwife at 36 weeks. This entails bending the knees and seeing how far apart the mother can open her knees without pain (Figure 12.3).

It is vital that all care givers in labour are aware of this measurement and understand the implications for birth.

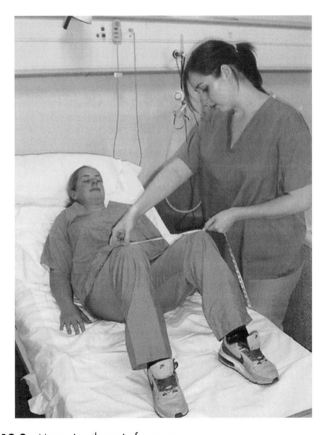

Figure 12.3 Measuring the pain-free gap.

Intrapartum care

Case study 12.2 Birth story: elective caesarean section and PGP

Michelle started to feel pain in the region of her symphysis pubis at about 30 weeks. She was told by her midwife that it was just the baby moving down, a warm bath would help and it would all resolve when the baby was born! I first met Michelle on the postnatal ward. She had given birth with the aid of a Ventouse 2 days earlier. Michelle was experiencing severe pain and having difficulty moving.

Baby care, including feeding her baby, was almost impossible. Both Michelle and her partner were unhappy with their care. Codeine and paracetamol were insufficient to control her pain and her immobility was reducing her ability to care for herself and the baby. She was becoming very distressed.

I asked Michelle to describe her pain and whether any particular movements exacerbated the pain or made it better. I then asked her to show me the range of mobility she had in her legs and hips. All her signs and symptoms pointed to the fact that Michelle was suffering from PGP. I arranged for an obstetric physiotherapist and the pain team nurse to visit and set up a management programme for her. Locally designed written information was given to Michelle and contact details for the NCT were also made available.

It was nearly 2 years later when I next met Michelle as she was booking into hospital for an elective caesarean section. During the preceding years, she had spent a great deal of time finding out about PGP. Her symptoms had resolved eventually, although not totally until 6 months postpartum. In this second pregnancy, the symptoms had reappeared at 28 weeks. This time Michelle was better prepared and had been treated by an osteopath. She was on crutches but remained mobile. Michelle had discussed her labour options and had decided to opt for an elective caesarean section, rather than going through labour and risking another assisted birth in the lithotomy position.

It may seem obvious but it is vital that birth companions are aware of the mother's mobility and any limitations. The pain-free knee gap should be recorded in the birth plan, and the birth companion needs to be aware of how wide that gap is in practice (Figure 12.4). It is a good idea to find out which positions work well for the woman by trying them out at home first. Positions that are impractical need to be highlighted in the birth plan as potential problems (Case study 12.2).

As with any other choices during labour, birth companions may need to act as an advocate for the woman, functioning as an effective link between the woman and health professionals.

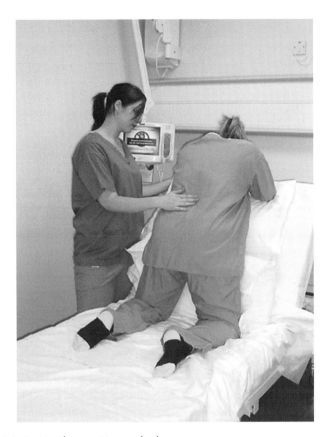

Figure 12.4 Kneeling position on bed.

Pain relief in labour

There is no reason why a woman should not choose any of the options available for managing her pain in labour. Some women may have already used TENS during the antenatal period for localised relief of pain. If she hasn't used TENS before this is a good locally focused pain option that the woman can be shown how to use at home before she goes into labour.

There is some debate about whether hydrotherapy is a good choice for mothers with PGP. The benefits of free mobility and buoyancy need to be weighed against the movement of entering and standing in the pool (Figure 12.5). This should be discussed with the woman and her therapists (physiotherapist, osteopath, etc.) and it is usually worthwhile asking her to establish whether she can enter the pool unassisted by visiting the intended place of birth. In hospitals or birthing units where a hoist is available, women will still be able leave the pool readily in an emergency.

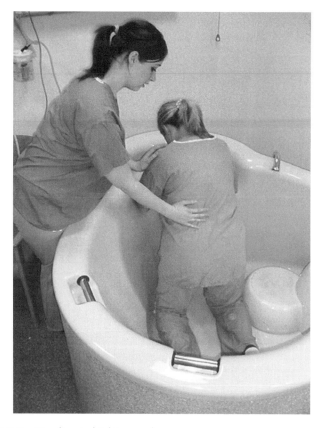

Figure 12.5 Kneeling in birthing pool.

Many women with PGP will have already used complementary therapies during the antenatal period and found them effective. Most complementary therapies are suitable during labour, but difficulties may centre on access to appropriately trained midwives or complementary therapists who are able to treat a woman in labour. This is particularly difficult in hospitals or birthing units where trusts are unable to offer vicarious liability. In the mother's own home she may choose a practitioner who is available throughout her labour.

Midwives should remember their code of practice regarding their role in relation to the use of complementary therapies without appropriate qualifications (NMC, 2004). Useful information about using complementary methods in conjunction with mainstream midwifery care is available from Denise Tiran's website at www.expectancy.co.uk.

There doesn't appear to be any contra-indication to the use of intramuscular injections of pethidine or meptazinol for women with PGP. The only caution relates to mobility and positioning if mother is disoriented by the use of opiates.

Epidurals do have the potential to cause harm if posture and mobility are compromised by a 'heavy' epidural. It is very important that the woman's legs are well supported and not allowed to 'fall apart'. The so-called low dose 'mobile' epidural does reduce the likelihood of poor positioning in bed, improves mobility during a long labour and is helpful during invasive procedures such as vaginal examination or fetal blood sampling.

Positions for labour and birth

Some women with PGP decide that the best option for them is an elective caesarean section, especially if they have had problems during a previous labour and birth. However, as with any elective section it is important that the midwife offers the woman clear information relating to the pros and cons of a major surgical operation.

Women planning for a vaginal birth should be given the opportunity to try different positions in their chosen place of birth, i.e. home, hospital or birth centre. This is a good time to measure the pain-free knee gap, try a dry run into and out of the pool and to explore the most comfortable positions for use on the bed or birthing ball (Figure 12.6).

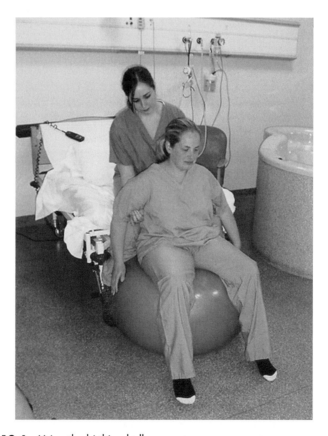

Figure 12.6 Using the birthing ball.

Kneeling may be possible using bean bags or pillows and it has the added advantage of utilising gravity. This position is also really good for vaginal examinations. The left lateral position may or may not reduce strain on the pelvis. If the woman does want to try left lateral it is vital that her top leg is supported by a bed table or lithotomy supports padded with pillows (Figure 12.7). This should prevent over abduction of the hips.

Remember that the comfort level of previously tried and tested positions may alter by the time the labour commences. Previous plans may need to be adapted or altered completely. Most straddling positions are not comfortable during labour, so sitting on the birthing ball or pushing on the toilet are probably not the best options. However, the midwife should be led by the woman who is the best judge of the limits of her mobility.

The biggest danger and potential for injury during labour is associated with the traditional use of lithotomy poles and supports. It is

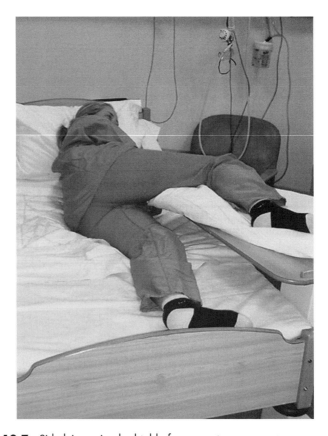

Figure 12.7 Side lying using bed table for support.

important that both legs are lifted up together to minimise the gap between the knees and limit abduction of the hips. When lifting the legs into position they need to be well supported, particularly when an epidural is in place. There are times when the use of lithotomy poles is required for instrumental delivery or suturing but it is vital to maintain an awareness of the pain-free gap in order to prevent any injury that might have long-term effects. Fetal blood sampling is often performed in the lithotomy position but the NICE guidelines for intrapartum monitoring (NICE, 2007) do recommend the left lateral position for this procedure (Figure 12.8). The midwife should take the initiative to ensure that women only remain in the lithotomy position for the minimum amount of time that is really required.

A final concern is the practice of placing a woman's feet on midwives' hips. This is not only poor practice that can be harmful for the woman in labour but it is also bad for the midwives' posture (Case study 12.3).

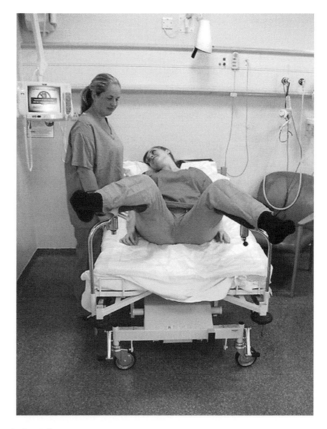

Figure 12.8 Lithotomy position.

Case study 12.3 Birth story: water birth and PGP

Caroline had experienced PGP with her first pregnancy and during labour felt that she had continually retold her midwife what she was and was not able to do during labour. Although she delivered vaginally, she had an epidural in labour and gave birth to her baby in a semi-recumbent position on the bed. With her second pregnancy Caroline had been in touch with the SPD association and gained valuable information to help her plan for this pregnancy and labour. By the time I was in contact with Caroline she was on crutches, had limited mobility and was seriously debating about having an elective LSCS. We discussed her options for both analgesia and birth. She had heard that water may help because it encourages mobility, buoyancy and allows freedom to move unassisted. The biggest concern related to Caroline's ability to enter the pool unassisted (although her local unit did have a hoist it was for emergency use only) and whether she would be able to stand if an emergency did occur.

As part of her plan of care Caroline attended the hospital in the later stages of pregnancy where she discovered that she was able to get in and out of the pool unassisted.

I was on duty when Caroline went into labour. The labour was induced and Caroline was worried that she wouldn't be able to use the pool after all. But because the induction was with prostin (and all other parameters were normal) there was no contra-indication to using the pool. Caroline proceeded to get into the water, where she had a rapid labour and water birth followed by a 6-hour transfer back home. The postnatal period was uneventful for both her and the baby.

The birth stories have been included in this chapter to highlight the fact that there is no right or wrong answer for labour and birth. Preferences should be discussed, options highlighted, professional advice sought (from traditional and/or complementary therapists) and a birth plan designed to offer the widest range of choices possible.

Postnatal care – mobility or bed rest?

Mens et al. (1996) has some wise words for the postnatal period: 'It is important to slowly start working on improving your condition. During your pregnancy certain activities had to be slowly run down, and afterwards it is best to gradually build them up again'. After the birth of the baby, it is just as important as it was during pregnancy for midwives to continue listening to women and encourage them to work with their own bodies.

Some women will benefit from bed rest for 24–48 hours until pain subsides. A wheelchair can be used for trips to the bathroom. Many women will need assistance with feeding and baby care, especially when lifting baby out of the cot.

If a woman is on bed rest, encourage her to do postnatal exercises regularly to avoid deep vein thrombosis. Anti-embolism stockings and prophylactic low molecular weight heparin are strongly advised if the period of bed rest is greater than 24 hours (Lewis, 2001). The best time to commence gradual mobilisation is when the woman feels ready and it should progress within the limits of her experience of the pain.

Analgesia

The need for pain relief can range from the use of paracetamol or TENS, to stronger preparations such as opiates and anti-inflammatories. The pain clinic team (who unfortunately often have long waiting lists) may be able to offer effective local or regional anaesthesia. It is worth trying to organise an appointment or referral whilst still in hospital.

Complementary therapists can also offer alternatives to the medical management of pain if the woman wishes. Many women will be keen to continue the use of therapies that have been helpful to them during the pregnancy.

Continuing support

The input provided in pregnancy from specialists, such as physiotherapists, occupational therapists, health visitors and social services, should follow on seamlessly after the birth of the baby. A plan of care should be in place prior to discharge from hospital or birth centre to home.

Family and support group involvement needs to continue too. It has been suggested that it may take 3–12 months to recover from PGP and women will want to take this into consideration if and when they plan their next pregnancy.

For a small number of women, the recovery time will be prolonged beyond 12 months after the birth of the baby and referral to orthopaedic specialists will become a necessity. Literature, relating to PGP generally, suggests that one little-known treatment option is prolotherapy. Franke (2003) states that evaluation should view the pelvis as a whole and consider all of its six articulations. A biomechanical assessment can then identify whether mobilisation or stabilisation is required to bring the pelvis back into alignment. Stabilisation exercises and belts or taping are the first steps in the treatment programme, but if these fail to maintain stabilisation then prolotherapy can be considered. Prolotherapy increases joint stabilisation and is used widely in the field of sports medicine. It has been used for many years to stabilise the sacroiliac joints of those with severe lower back pain with little evidence of adverse side effects (Ongley et al., 1987). A solution of glucose/dextrose is injected into the osseoligamentous junctions of the targeted pelvic joint. The solution is an irritant that dehydrates the tissues to cause severe local damage. An inflammatory reaction follows that attracts fibroblasts, which subsequently lay down new collagen fibres to strengthen the ligament. The process is impeded by anti-inflammatory drugs such as aspirin or NSAIDS (Fonstad, 2005).

In very rare circumstances women are referred to an orthopaedic surgeon, where the symphysis pubis is fused, wired or plated. However, there is little research on this ultimate management, with the European Commission commenting that 'randomized trials are needed to establish the effect of fusion surgery in PGP patients not responding to non-operative treatment' (Vleeming et al., 2004).

Reoccurrence

The exact rate of reoccurrence is unclear but it has been reported that as many as 85% of women will experience PGP again with their next pregnancy. Leadbetter et al. (2004) also suggest that 53–72% of women with PGP during pregnancy will find that symptoms reoccur when menstruation starts again. The effects of breastfeeding are unclear and may or may not exacerbate symptoms.

Women with a history of pre-menstrual syndrome are likely to have pre-menstrual pelvic pain. When the need arises to begin using contraception again, women who have experienced PGP should be made aware that oral, injectable and implant methods can cause pelvic pain to return, due to changes in levels of progesterone. In the longer term, women who use hormone replacement therapy may find that pelvic pain is aggravated or returns. Consideration of these issues would appear to support the strong hormonal theory associated with PGP.

Summary

Supporting women with PGP is a challenge for community midwives. Women living with this difficult condition require extensive physical and psychological support. It is vital that midwives work in partnership with other health professionals, both traditional and complementary, so that the care women experience is effective.

A woman will feel the benefit of loving support from family, friends, support groups and professionals who understand her limitations. They can help her to implement strategies that enhance her ability to negotiate normal daily activities and achieve an emotionally fulfilling birth experience. At the heart of care are empathy, understanding, knowledge and the willingness to tackle what is still a relatively misunderstood condition.

> ### Key points
>
> - Pelvic girdle pain is the accepted terminology for the condition previously known as symphysis pubis dysfunction.
> - Teamwork and appropriate referral to health professionals, social services and complementary therapists will support women in meeting the challenges of living with PGP.
> - Birth plans are a useful tool for planning care and communicating vital information about the woman's physical limitations and aspirations for birth.
> - Family, friends and support groups have a vital role in psychosocial support.

Acknowledgement

Dianne would like to thank the students of University of Greenwich and Darent Valley Hospital, Kent who contributed to the photographs, and the mothers who have shared their experiences and birth stories.

Sources of information and support

Association of Chartered Physiotherapists in Women's Health
c/o Chartered Society of Physiotherapists
14 Bedford Row
London
WC1R 4ED

British DSP Support Group
www.spd-uk.org

Expectant Parent Complementary Therapies Consultancy
www.expectancy.co.uk

The Pelvic Partnership
This comprehensive website was created by people who have experienced PGP.

www.pelvicpartnership.org.uk

References

ACPWHealth (1996) *Symphysis Pubis Dysfunction*. Association of Chartered Physiotherapists in Women's Health, London.

Albert, H., Godskesen, M., Westergaard, J. (2000) Evaluation of clinical tests used in classification procedures in pregnancy related pelvic joint pain. *European Spine Journal*, **9**, 161–166.

Andrew, C. (2005) *The Role of Chiropractic in the Treatment of Symphysis Pubis Dysfunction/Pelvic Girdle Pain*. Oral presentation, ICM, Brisbane Australia.

Depledge, J., McNair, P.J., Keal-Smith, C. and Williams, M. (2005) Management of symphysis pubis dysfunction during pregnancy using exercise and pelvic support belts. *Physical Therapy*, **85**, 12.

Elden, H., Ladfors, L., Olsen, M.F., Ostgaard, H.C. and Hagberg, H. (2005) Effects of acupuncture and stabilising exercises as adjunct to standard treatment in pregnant women with pelvic girdle pain: randomised single blind controlled trial. *British Medical Journal*, **330** (7494), 761.

Fonstad, P. (2005) Prolotherapy in the treatment of low back pain: a literature review. *Journal of Manual and Manipulative Therapy*, **13** (1), 27–34.

Franke, B.A. (2003) Formative dynamics: the pelvic girdle. *Journal of Manual and Manipulative Therapy*, **11** (1), 12–40.

Hollingworth, J. and Hawley, J.H. (1994) Severe vitamin D deficiency in pregnancy. *Journal of Obstetrics and Gynaecology*, **14** (6), 430–431.

HSE (2007) MSD return to work – Agreeing a return to work plan, Health and Safety Executive, http://www.hse.gov.uk/sicknessabscence/msd.htm (accessed 13.11.07).

Kristiansson, P., Svardsudd, K. and Schoultz, B. (1996) Serum relaxin, symphyseal pain and back pain during pregnancy. *American Journal of Obstetrics and Gynaecology*, **175**, 1342–1347.

Leadbetter, R.E., Mawer, D. and Lindow, S.W. (2004) Symphysis pubis dysfunction: a review of the literature. *Journal of Maternal Fetal and Neonatal Medicine*, **16** (6), 349–356.

Lewis, G. (ed) (2001) *Why Mothers Die – Confidential Enquiry into Maternal Deaths 1997–1999*. RCOG Press, London.

Mens, J.M., Vleeming, A., Stoeckart, R. et al. (1996) Understanding peripartum pelvic pain. Implications of a patient survey. *Spine*, **21**, 1363–1369.

Mens, J.M., Vleeming, A., Snijders, C.J., Koes, B.W. and Stam, H.J. (2001) Reliability and validity of the active straight leg raise test in posterior pelvic pain since pregnancy. *Spine* **26**, 1167–1171.

NICE (2007) *Intrapartum care: Care of healthy women and their babies during childbirth*, National Institute for Health and Clinical Excellence, London.

NMC (2004) *Midwives Rules and Standards*. Nursing and Midwifery Council, London.

Ongley, M.J., Klein, R.G., Dorman, T.A., Eek, B.C. and Hubert, L.J. (1987) A new approach to the treatment of chronic low back pain. *Lancet*, July 18, 143–146.

Ostgaard, H.C., Zetherstrom, G., Roos-Hansson, E. and Svanberg, B. (1994) Reduction in back and posterior pelvic pain in pregnancy. *Spine* **19** (8), 894–900.

Shepherd, J. (2005) Symphysis pubis dysfunction: a hidden cause of morbidity. *British Journal of Midwifery*, **13** (5), 301–307.

Vangen, S., Stoltenberg, C. and Stray-Pedersen, B. (1999) Complaints and complications in pregnancy: a study of ethnic Norwegian and ethnic Pakistan women in Oslo. *Ethnicity and Health*, **4** (1/2), 19–28.

Vleeming, A., Albert, H.B., van der Helm, F.C.T., Lee, D., Östgaard, H.C., Stuge, B. and Sturesson, B. (2004) A definition of joint stability. In: *European Guidelines on the Diagnosis and Treatment of Pelvic Girdle Pain. Cost Action B13; Low Back Pain: Guidelines for its Management.* Working group 4, European Commission, Brussels.

Wedenberg, K., Berit, M. and Norling, A. (2000) A prospective randomized study comparing acupuncture with physiotherapy for low back and pelvic pain in pregnancy. *Acta obstetricia et gynecologica Scandinavica*, **79**, 331–335.

Wellock, V. (2002) The ever widening gap – symphysis pubis dysfunction. *British Journal of Midwifery*, **10** (6), 348–353.

Wellock, V.K., Crichton, M.A. and McGowen, L. (2005) *Understanding Pregnant Women's Perceptions of Symphysis Pubis Dysfunction.* Oral presentation, ICM, Brisbane.

Index